A I D S

And Its Treatment
by
Traditional Chinese Medicine

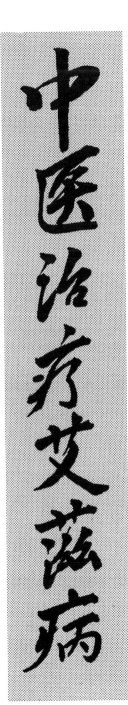

A I D S

And
Its Treatment by
T r a d i t i o n a l
Chinese Medicine

Chief Chinese Editor:
Huang Bing-shan

Compilers:
Huang Bing-shan
He Yu-zin
Sun Qian
Ma Dong-xin
Zhang Xiao-wei
Han Yu-shan
Wang Go-en
Zhang Jian
Lu Yan
Brian MacKenna

Consultant:
Cong Zhong

Translators:
Fu Di & Bob Flaws

Published by:

BLUE POPPY PRESS, INC.
1775 LINDEN AVE.
BOULDER, CO 80304

First Edition, November, 1991
Second Printing, April, 1996

ISBN 0-936185-28-7
LC 91-73953

COMP Designation: A functional translation using a standard translational terminology

Printed at C & M Press in Denver, CO on recycled paper

10 9 8 7 6 5 4 3

Preface

by Bob Flaws

AIDS & Its Treatment by Traditional Chinese Medicine is a specially prepared English edition of *Zhong Yi Zhi Liao Ai Zi Bing* compiled under the guidance of Huang Bing-shan, Vice President of the Heilongjiang College of TCM in Harbin, PRC. The Chinese version of this book was published in Harbin by the Heilongjiang Science & Technology Press in 1990. In the last couple of years, many Western TCM practitioners have met Dr. Huang both in China and during his teaching tours to the West. Dr. Huang has made great efforts in spreading the benefits of TCM to the rest of the world by his openness and hospitality in hosting foreign students at the Heilongjiang College of TCM and by his assembly of a cadre of researchers and translators at that college engaged in the preparation of a number of books on TCM specifically for English-speaking practitioners. Those who know Dr. Huang appreciate his humor, candor, and straightforwardness as much as his profound knowledge of TCM.

This English language edition of *Zhong Yi Zhi Liao Ai Zi Bing* is a translation of the Chinese original to which additions and

revisions have been made. These changes have been made both to expand and update the material and to make this material more accessible to Western practitioners. TCM in Chinese is stated in a very codified and systematic technical language. Compared to most Western writing, it is formulaic in structure and highly syllogistic. Each sentence is part of a logical progression expressed in pithy and terse technical language which is often difficult to render in English. The original translation was prepared in Harbin by Fu Di, a translator attached to the college there. Fu Di was assisted by Stephen Oakley, an American studying at the college. The Chinese original and this working English language translation were then passed to me for retranslation and editing.

Because this book will be primarily used by Western practitioners of TCM in their clinical treatment of AIDS patients and others suffering from chronic, virally induced, immune deficiency disorders, such as CFIDS, we have striven to stay as close to the Chinese original as possible. We have adopted much of slational terminology suggested by Nigel Wiseman in *Glossary of Chinese Medical Terms and Acupuncture Points,* Paradigm Publications, Brookline, MA, 1990. We have tried to render a consistent translation and not just a paraphrase or gloss since it is our belief that the precision and logic of TCM is often lost in translation if that translation becomes too loose. Unfortunately, I did not have access to the Chinese original of several of the short sections added to this English language edition. In these cases, I have simply edited the best I could.

As stated above, the language and literature of TCM is highly stylized and very compact. Chinese as a language packs a great deal of meaning and import into only a few words. Because of its staccato nature lacking most of the grammar of Western languages, the many connotations of a single word often intentionally color the use of that word deepening the meaning implied but not explicitly and exhaustively stated. One of the mistakes many Chinese translators make is that they try to make the TCM literature sound like modern Western medical literature. This, I believe, is a great mistake. It typically obscures the technical meaning and logic of the Chinese original. It may sound better to non-TCM Western medical practitioners, but it does not accurately convey the meaning and methodology of TCM. Therefore, I believe it is extremely important for English language translators of TCM to stick as closely to the Chinese as possible. I also agree with Nigel Wiseman that this further means the creation of a technical TCM terminology in English which, as a technical vocabulary, will sound a bit strange to laypersons.

As I have also stated elsewhere, I believe that it is very important for all Western schools and colleges of TCM to teach and require the study of medical Chinese. It is far easier to understand TCM in Chinese than in translation. As an extension of this, I do not think that an English translation must expunge all Chinese words. Therefore, in this translation, we have retained a host of Chinese technical terms. In most cases, we give both the Chinese and its translation. However, if the word or compound phrase appears repeatedly, we have not felt the need to translate it every time. There are a host of TCM technical terms which should simply be incorporated into our English TCM vocabulary. Some words' and terms' use is so repeated and pervasive in TCM, they should not require translation.

As an extension of this, I would draw the reader's special attention to the first two chapters of this book. These are the introductory chapters concerning the TCM categorization of AIDS, its TCM etiology and pathophysiology, and its basic TCM treatment principles. TCM is a rational style of medicine based on theory as well as on empirical experience. The practice of TCM is as much a function of thinking in terms of this theory as it is the rote memorization of treatment protocols. If one understands the import and implications of this introductory theory as it applies to AIDS, one will be able to apply the treatments given in this book all the more successfully. Therefore, I recommend clinicians to not skip over this material and rush to the formulas listed for various disease conditions but to read these theoretical sections sentence by sentence searching for the logic behind each statement and their deeper implications. As an editor and translator, it is my job to look at each word in each sentence and each sentence in each paragraph to see their logical connection and necessity. If I have learned anything about TCM in the past dozen years, it is largely because of such close reading of a number of TCM texts.

This is the first Blue Poppy publication where we have given both the latinate pharmacological identification of medicinals in formulas and their *pinyin*. We hope this makes the process of identification easier for readers. We have based our identifications on Bensky & Gamble's *Chinese Herbal Medicine: Materia Medica*; Hong-yen Hsu's *Oriental Materia Medica: A Concise Guide*; Cloudburst Press' *A Barefoot Doctor's Manual*; and Southern Material Center's *Chinese Materia Medica*, Vol. 1-6, published in Taipei. Acupuncture point identifications for channel points are given both in *pinyin* and according to the numbering system found in *Essentials of Chinese Acupuncture*. Extra-channel points are identified in *pinyin* and according to the numbering system in *Acupuncture: A Comprehensive Text*.

This book has been compiled by a team of researchers. The Chinese original shows a number of different styles of wording and phrasing. We have not endeavored to change this. Chapter 7, Section 3 in the Chinese original consists of a rather long list of formulas categorized as either supporting the righteous and consolidating the root, clearing heat and resolving toxins, activating the blood and transforming stasis, softening the hard and scattering nodulation, and others, meaning miscellaneous. Under each formula there is a listing of its ingredients, TCM functions, and indications. The majority of these formulas have already been discussed in the preceding chapters under the treatment of various pathoconditions addressed. Since these formulas are all well known, standard ones, and since their ingredients, explanations, and modifications are all covered even more extensively in Bensky & Barolet's *Chinese Herbal Medicine: Formulas & Strategies*, we have chosen to only list these formulas with a brief mention of their major TCM indications. We have done this to both conserve trees, paper, and energy and also to keep the cost of this book down. All professional practitioners of TCM are expected to already be familiar with most of these formulas.

One of the strong points of this book is that it relies primarily on TCM's best known, standard prescriptions as guiding formulas. Likewise, it recommends only well known, standard acupuncture/moxibustion points. This makes this book all the more immediately usable since it bases treatment on what should be already known and understood protocols.

The weakest part of this book, from a Western point of view is, I think, its chapter on prevention and nursing. This chapter is very Chinese. It shows a certain naivete *vis a vis* homosexuality. Modern Chinese culture is very bourgeois, opinionated, conservative, and moralistic. We hope readers will not judge the validity of the treatments contained herein in the light of this chapter.

Because this book was written as a clinical manual for TCM practitioners, much of the information in this chapter on prevention and nursing seems scanty and abbreviated. This is because Chinese doctors are expected to be able to extrapolate both theoretically and practically from such technical code terms as "cold and raw", "hot and spicy", and "light" foods. Readers interested in further explanations of these dietary and lifestyle concepts should see *Chinese Medicated Diet* by Zhang Wen-gao *et al.* (Shanghai College of TCM Press), *Health Preservation and Rehabilitation* by Sun Guang-ren *et al.* (Shanghai College of TCM Press), *Prince Wen Hui's Cook: Chinese Dietary Therapy,* by myself and Honora Lee Wolfe (Paradigm Publications), and my *Nine Ounces: A Nine Part Program for the Prevention of AIDS in HIV Positive Persons,* and *Arisal of the Clear: A Simple Guide the Healthy Eating According to Traditional Chinese Medicine* (both published by Blue Poppy Press).

It was also thought to append a brief chapter on self-treatment to this English language edition. This would mainly have contained several *qi gong* exercises and a short *tai qi quan* form. Since the instructions for these did not contain any illustrations and since especially the *tai qi* cannot be learned solely from written instructions, we have decided not to include such a section. As stated above, this book is primarily meant as a clinical manual for practicing professionals. It is not intended for nor do we endorse self-treatment from this book by laypersons. We have suggested to Dr. Haung that his team compile such a self-help manual specifically for patients. In the meantime HIV positives and PWA's should be encouraged to take classes in and practice *qi gong* and *tai qi.* Instruction in these arts is available in most urban centers in the Western world.

In 1989, I wrote a slim little book called *Nine Ounces: A Nine Part Program for the Prevention of AIDS in HIV Positive Persons*. This book is both a theoretical discussion of the TCM categorization and etiology of AIDS and various self-help therapies logically derived from that discussion. In *Nine Ounces*, I identified AIDS as a species of *wen bing* or warm disease due to pestilential evils or *yi xie* which could also be categorized as *fu wen xie* or hidden warm evils which enter the *xue fen* or blood phase first and work their way from the lower burner upwards to the upper burner and from the inside to the outside. This TCM categorization of AIDS was based on a short article by Wu Bo-ping and Lu Shou-kang appearing in the now defunct *Journal of the American College of TCM* in 1987 and my own further thought on the line of logic suggested by Wu and Lu. Two years later, it is gratifying to see that such eminent TCM scholars and authorities as Dr. Huang and his associates corroborate and substantiate this same opinion. As Dr. Huang *et al.* demonstrate, once one makes this identification, it has many implications for the TCM diagnosis, prognosis, and treatment of AIDS.

This book does not purport to offer *the* cure for AIDS. As yet, there is no completely satisfactory cure for this devastating epidemic disease. However, TCM treatment is able to improve many AIDS patients' immunity. It is able to keep asymptomatic HIV positive patients asymptomatic for long periods of time if not indefinitely. It is able to back off the symptoms of most ARC patients, returning many to asymptomatic carrier status. And it can often significantly help treat, control, and eliminate many of the opportunistic infections associated with full blown AIDS. However, such ability is not the function of a particular herb or formula but is based on the rational methodology of TCM which treats not only the disease but the individual patient as a whole.

I have been treating AIDS patients with TCM since 1982. I have been consciously basing my treatments on the categorization of AIDS as a *wen bing* due to a *fu wen xie* since 1987 when I came across Wu and Lu's article in the *JACTCM*. However, in the last six months or so since gaining access to this book, I must also say that I have found the differential diagnosis and formulas it contains to be particularly effective. This book is easy to use, clear, and systematic. I believe it will be of great benefit to English speaking practitioners of TCM and the AIDS patients they serve.

I would like to add a note of caution concerning the internal administration of the herbal formulas given in this book. These should only be prescribed by professional practitioners specifically trained in TCM *nei ke* or internal medicine, *ben cao* or materia medica, and *fang ji xue* or the writing of prescriptions. The prescription of internal medicine requires a higher degree of training and competence than does the practice of acupuncture/moxibustion because it is more liable to cause side effects and iatrogenesis if misprescribed. Chinese medicinals are only safe and benign when prescribed correctly. When erroneously prescribed, they are just as likely to cause ill effects as modern Western drugs. Prescriptions and their ingredients given in this book are only meant as a guide or reference. In almost every case, the words *jia wei* or *jia jian* are appended to formula names. This means that the formula is meant to be prescribed with additions or additions and subtractions, *i.e.*, modifications depending upon the idiosyncracies of each presenting patient. These formulas should not be prescribed by rote unless the patient's signs and symptoms exactly tally with the those given in the clinical manifestations section. The treatment of AIDS patients is not the place to be learning the practice of internal medicine.

Not all practitioners feel up to the treatment of AIDS. I sincerely applaud those practitioners who chose not to treat AIDS patients based on a recognition that their knowledge and experience are not commensurate to the demands of this dangerous and complex disease. However, even those practitioners who do not have any HIV patients will find much useful information in this book. Other viral diseases may also be categorized as *wen bing* due to the internal invasion of hidden warm evils. For instance, I have found the theoretical discussions of the etiology and pathophysiology of the lymphadenopathy, which typically accompanies chronic immune deficiency fatigue syndrome (CFIDS), and the formulas for its treatment given in this book to be very helpful in treating that symptom in CFIDS patients. Modern Western medical research is beginning to suspect that a large number of diseases may be due to viral invasion and its attendant depression in immune function, such as lupus, cancer, and even diabetes just to name a few. If this is so, I believe this book may also shed light on the TCM treatment of those diseases as well.

I applaud Dr. Huang and his associates and graduate students at the Heilongjiang College of TCM for preparing this text and others with Western practitioners of TCM in mind. Now it is up to us Western practitioners of TCM to study these and similar texts and to upgrade our understanding and practice of the unique, rational, and wise methodology of TCM.

Foreword

by Huang Bing-shan

AIDS is a new kind of epidemic disease in the world today. As of this writing, AIDS has spread rapidly to every continent of the world. It is a very fatal disease with a high death rate amongst those infected. It has been cursed as "the new epidemic of the 80s" and is sometimes referred to as "supercancer". It is also one of those medical problems which human beings have yet to solve. At present, systematic, worldwide research is being conducted on this topic. However, as of yet, modern Western medicine has not discovered any totally satisfactory and effective treatments for this disease.

Traditional Chinese Medicine (TCM) has accumulated several thousand years of experience in the prevention and treatment of disease. Many research studies have shown that Chinese medicine is able to improve the body's immunity and inhibit viruses. Based on these well established facts, the treatment and prevention of AIDS with Chinese medicine has drawn increasingly more attention from researchers both in and out of China. In recent years, we have been cooperating with various scientific research institutes abroad and have tried to treat AIDS with Chinese medicine. Some encouraging results have been achieved and the principles of diagnosing and treating AIDS with TCM have, I believe, been established. This book has, therefore, been written to promote the study of treating and preventing AIDS with Traditional Chinese Medicine. In this book, we have outlined the TCM method of treating AIDS with herbal medicine, acupuncture, diet, and lifestyle modifications. This is all based on our clinical experience and the rational theories of TCM. We have also included related information from both TCM and modern Western medicine to make these dicussions more detailed and precise.

We hope this book may serve as a handy reference for those researchers and clinicians in the field of AIDS. Because of our haste in writing and translating this book, there may be some mistakes contained herein. We hope our colleagues and peers will point these out to us.

In the course of compiling this book, some of my fellow students, An Xue-mei, Yin Yan, Wang Jing-bo, Meng Fan-bin, Wu Yue-xin, Chen Qan, Qi Shan, Jia Chun-bao, Zhang Bao-wen, and Wang Yuan-hong, helped me in classifying and collating the materials collected. Fu Di translated and edited the entire book in China. Mr. Stephen Oakley also helped in China to check the English grammar. And Cong Zhong acted as a most appreciated consultant. I would like to express my gratitude and appreciation to all these kind helpers.

Contents

6

1

Introduction

AIDS is an acronym for acquired immune deficiency syndrome. This is a breakdown in human immunity caused by the human immune virus (HIV) resulting in a clinical syndrome of numerous opportunistic infections and cancers. It is a new type of infectious disease which is drawing great attention. The disease has spread very quickly and is widespread. So far, it has covered all 5 continents with a death rate in excess of 50% in some locations. AIDS has been called "supercancer" and a "world wide epidemic disease". Its damage greatly threatens the health of the human race. Though exhaustive research in countries all over the world has resulted in the development of over 100 kinds of synthetic drugs, these treatments have not proven effective. The prospect of the development of an AIDS vaccine is exciting, but unfortunately there has not been much progress on that front. Meanwhile, researchers and clinicians abroad experienced in Traditional Chinese Medicine have made some encouraging achievements in treating AIDS with TCM. The following is a description of the current state of the art in the treatment of AIDS with both Western medicine and TCM.

Modern Western Medicine & AIDS

I. Epidemiology

A. Current Status of the AIDS Epidemic Worldwide

The disease was first reported in America in June 1981. Prior to that, the first reported cases of Kaposi's sarcoma and *Pneumocystis carinii* pneumonia occurred in the United States in 1978 and '79 respectively. Evidence later indicated that these diseases are related to an acquired deficiency of immunocytes. In 1982, AIDS became the officially adopted acronym for this acquired immune deficiency syndrome. After 6 years of researching case histories, the American Tumor Research Institute has proven that the AIDS virus originated in central Africa. Its first incidence appeared in Zaire and spread to other countries in central Africa. Subsequent to this outbreak, the virus spread to Haiti in the Caribbean. In the late 1970s, American homosexuals carried the virus to America.

Since the 1980s, AIDS has spread violently in America, Europe, and Oceana (*i.e.* Australia, New Zealand) and especially in technologically developed, industrial countries. AIDS has ravaged a number of countries in Africa. There is some incidence of AIDS in South America and the virus has finally reached Asia. The World Health Organization (WHO) gave statistical estimates in 1982. At that time, only 711 cases had been reported in 16 countries. By the end of 1985, the reports indicated 17,073 cases in 68 countries and in 1986, more than 32,590 cases in 101 countries. Since 1985, the incidence of AIDS in the United States has doubled each year. By June 1987, there had been 52,602 cases reported in 118 countries with a clear tendency of continued proliferation. As of Nov. 1, 1988, AIDS had increased to a total of 124,114 cases in 142 countries of which 29,861 cases were reported in 1988 alone. As of Dec. 1, 1990, WHO has reported a worldwide incidence of 307,000 cases of which some 50,000 were reported in the United States.

At present, the number of cases of this fierce epidemic is still spreading worldwide with infected patients increasing constantly. By Dec. 1, 1989, 152 countries had reported some 190,000 cases to the Global Planning Department of WHO. The Americas are responsible for 71% of this number, the U.S. having the majority of cases with Brazil and Canada also accounting for high percentages. Europe is responsible for 12% and Africa for 16%, while Asia had the least incidence of all the continents. Most Asian patients, mainly Japanese, were infected after injecting imported blood products.

The Chinese Ministry of Health reported 32 cases on Dec. 1, 1990. By Feb. 8, 1990, the number of patients infected with AIDS in the PRC had increased rapidly to 194 cases among which 146 cases were discovered while monitoring drug addicts in Yunnan Province. This rapid increase in number has created a very serious problem for Chinese medical workers. According to WHO's estimates, there will be 50-100 million AIDS virus carriers worldwide by the year 1991. Because there is no effective treatment or prevention, the death rate increases unabated. All these facts greatly alarm society evoking a sense of grave concern. AIDS has become an increasingly important public health issue facing countries all over the world.

B. Pathways of Transmission

AIDS is an infectious disease caused by a virus. The results of seroepidemiological research have shown that the AIDS virus is transmitted through blood, saliva, and sperm and across the placenta.

1. Sexual transmission

The extraction of the retrovirus from sperm has provided clear proof that the AIDS virus can be transmitted during sex. In some developed countries, such as the United States, homosexual activities cause injury to the sexual organs, rectal mucosa, and anus. Such injury provides an ideal biological condition for the invasion of the AIDS virus. In African countries, prostitutes are the main transmitters.

2. Blood transmission

It has been confirmed that blood and its products can transmit AIDS. This mainly refers to contamination of coagulation factor products introduced in the course of blood transfusions and especially affects those who depend on such products for a long period of time, such as hemophiliacs. In the case of drug users who frequently inject themselves, AIDS infection often results from the use of contaminated needles.

3. Mother-fetus transmission

Mother-fetus transmission is directly through the placenta. According to statistical evidence, 9% AIDS patients are women of childbearing age between 13-39 years old, and 20% of children with AIDS became infected in the womb. Therefore, extrapolating from the incidence of AIDS in women, we can predict the tendency of AIDS in the newborn children of AIDS-infected mothers.

4. Transmission by professional or incidental contact

Professional transmission is usually caused by needle stick or trauma whereby the integrity of the practitioner's skin is compromised and subsequently exposed to contaminated blood. Incidental transmission refers to common contact in the family. This kind of transmission poses little danger. However, this possibility does exist if the integrity of the skin is compromised and body fluids are exchanged.

AIDS may attack a number of very different kinds of people. Homosexuals, intravenous drug users, and hemophiliacs have the highest rates of infection with 250-350 in every 100,000 of such people. The rate of infection of those who receive blood transfusions is 0.6 and, among children, 2.8 in every 100,000. The rate of infection is relatively low in the American population at large at only 0.1 per 100,000. According to the Center for Disease Control statistics, AIDS mainly infects people under 45, the average age being 34, and predominantly males. Females represent only 7% of the total number of those infected. Sexual intercourse among heterosexuals shows an infection rate of only 0.8%. Distribution by race is as follows: Caucasians, 57%; Blacks, 26%; and Haitians, 12.9%.

II. AIDS Pathophysiology

In 1983, Luc Montagnier of the Pasteur Research Institute in Paris, France isolated a new kind of retrovirus (RV) from patients and named it lymphatic associated virus (LAV). Shortly afterwards in America, Robert Gallo also successfully isolated a new kind of RV which was later confirmed to be the AIDS virus. He named this the human T-lymphotrophic virus type III (HTLV III). At an international symposium on AIDS held in Paris in June 1986, this virus was officially named the human immune deficiency virus (HIV).

After invading the blood, this virus enters the subgroup of T_4 helper lymphocytes. Subsequent to the virus' invasion of these cells, it replicates and then releases more viruses into the bloodstream. This virus can also remain latent, in which case, the infected individual becomes an asymptomatic carrier. Patients during this latency period do not show any symptoms, but, under certain circumstances, can infect others and go on to develop the symptomatic stage. The reduction of T_4 cells leads to the relative increase of T_8 inhibitor lymphocytes with these two lymphocytes' normal proportions becoming reversed. At the same time, this inhibits antibody production. To make matters worse, this reversal in the proportion of T_4/T_8 and the immunodeficiency thus caused by the AIDS virus appears to be irreversible. This severe hypoimmunity allows for fatal opportunistic infections, such as *Pneumocystis carinii* pneumonia (PCP), and malignant tumors, such as Kaposi's sarcoma (KS).

Usually, the more particles the human T-lymphotrophic virus releases while replicating, the stronger the pathological effect the T-lymphocytes produce. As mentioned above, the target cells of the AIDS virus are the

T_4 cells. In the course of synthesis and multiplication of the AIDS virus, the normal T_4 cells are destroyed. Hence the body's immunity is compromised. This compromise is, unfortunately, the precursor to the symptomatic stage of AIDS. This vicious cycle—compromise-infection-further compromise-reinfection—describes the whole pathological course of this disease from the beginning stage of viral infection to the intermediate stage and, in time, to the development of full blown AIDS.

III. Clinical Manifestations

AIDS usually has a latency period varying from 6 months to 2-5 years. In the initial stage after infection, there is usually a short or transient symptomatic stage characterized by fatigue, fever, arthralgia, generalized lymphadenopathy, and/or diarrhea. After this, the patient tends to appear normal. Then, after an indeterminate dormant period, there may appear one or more varieties of clinical symptoms. For example, there may be fatigue, numbness of the limbs, tidal fever, night sweats, weight loss, reduced appetite, abdominal pain, diarrhea, or lymphadenopathy. Together, this group of symptoms is referred to as the AIDS-related complex (ARC). Later there may be rapid and sudden changes. These may include general changes in many systems and organs and multi-pathogen infections and complications. At present, based on clinical experience, the course of development of AIDS is usually divided into 3 periods or stages. The first stage is comprised of both the brief acute infection period and the asymptomatic latent period referred to together as the asymptomatic, antibody positive, virus-carrying stage. This stage may be overlooked due to an absence of symptoms. The second stage is the AIDS-related complex period or ARC. And the third stage is called full blown AIDS or advanced AIDS during which there are typically such complications as opportunistic infections and Kaposi's sarcoma.

A. Latent Stage AIDS

After the initial infection, there may be transient, generalized symptoms similar to those of nonspecific mononucleosis, such as fever, dizziness, sore throat, sweating, weakness, soreness in the joints, diarrhea, rash, and generalized lymphadenopathy. These symptoms usually last from 3-14 days. This is referred to as acute nonspecific viral syndrome. This is typically followed by an asymptomatic latency period of from 2-5 years with the average being 4 years. In some patients, this latency period may last even as long as 10-20 years.

B. AIDS-related Complex (ARC)

After the initial infection by the AIDS virus and its latent period, the patient may develop symptoms such as fever of unknown origin, lymphadenopathy, weight loss, diarrhea, thrush, and weakness. There may also be nonspecific complaints, such as apathy and depression or occasionally hyposexuality and impotence. The cause of these complaints and their relationship to AIDS remains unknown.

1. Fever

Fever is one of the most commonly encountered symptoms during the prodromal and ARC stages. It is usually due to unknown cause and is periodic, varying in degree from a prolonged, 38°C, low grade fever to an intermittent, 40°C, high fever. It is usually accompanied by general discomfort, weakness, night sweats, poor appetite, weight loss, and depression. Its causes are usually infection, malignant tumor, toxic reaction, allergic reaction, collagen disease, or autoimmune disease.

2. Diarrhea and weight loss

AIDS patients usually present with large amounts of watery diarrhea. This is typically a definite indication of opportunistic infections of the gastrointestinal tract or Kaposi's sarcoma. Progressive loss of body weight is also one of the early signs in some cases. Though eating and prolonged parenteral feeding are maintained, there is usually progressive cachexia. Body weight may be reduced by 20 or even 40%.

3. Skin lesions

AIDS or ARC patients may have skin rashes or itching. The rashes or lesions are usually diffuse, nonspecific maculopapulae. Other skin problems include progressive herpes mucosae, herpes simplex, and severe acute seborrheic dermatitis.

4. Generalized lymphadenopathy

Lymphadenopathy of unknown cause is also closely related to AIDS and is one of its clinical manifestations. Lymphadenopathy often lasts for over 3 months. It usually starts in the head or neck region and mainly involves the sternocleidomastoid lymph nodes. Lymphadenopathy may also come and go and is usually without tenderness. It may also sometimes be accompanied by weakness, intermittent low fever, night sweats, weight loss, and other systemic symptoms.

C. Full Blown AIDS

Patients in this stage are always extremely weak and emaciated with severely diminished immunity. They often exhibit severe opportunistic infections and malignant tumors, such as Kaposi's sarcoma.

1. Opportunistic infection

Pathogens causing opportunistic infection may be viral, bacterial, fungal, or parasitic and may appear throughout the body. Because of their virulent nature and thus the incurability of these infections, they are the main cause of death in AIDS patients. Infections may also be due to more than one pathogen at a time, causing polyinfections with complicated and unpredictable clinical manifestations.

One commonly seen opportunistic infection is *Pneumocystis carinii* pneumonia or PCP. After a long prodromal stage, patients may present with shortness of breath, dry cough, fever, and progressive dyspnea. The main pathological and clinical symptoms are confined to the lungs which show obvious disturbance in ventilation. Blood gas analysis tends to show hypoxemia and thoracography typically reveals localized or bilateral, diffuse infiltration spots indicative of interstitial pneumonia.

Toxoplasmosis often follows PCP. This is a commonly seen parasitic infection associated with AIDS which mainly attacks the central nervous system. Its manifestations include paralysis, localized nervous disorders, convulsions, disturbances in consciousness, and fever. It presents with a prolonged course of disease like that of meningitis or encephalitis. Physical examination usually reveals tumors. Therefore, this disease is easily discovered by pulmonary scan, computerized thermography (CT), or magnetic resonance imaging (MRI).

Another commonly seen disease associated with AIDS is oral candidiasis or thrush caused by *Candida albicans*. The affected area is typically very large. At the proximal end, it can cause erosion of the digestive tract resulting in dysphagia, odynophagia, and retrosternal burning pain. Other infectious pathogens include intestinal parasites, mycobacteria, cryptosporidia, cytomegalovirus, and herpes zoster virus.

2. Kaposi's sarcoma and other tumors

Kaposi's sarcoma or KS usually affects the skin, the mucosa, or the lymphatic system. Skin lesions are pink or red macular or papular eruptions. Their size varies from several millimeters to 1 centimeter. Other skin lesions are eruptions or carbuncles visible on the skin surface with a purple or brown color. These can develop quickly into tumors. They are usually surrounded by a ring of yellow-brown ecchymosis. In the early stage, there is no pain associated with these lesions. In the advanced stage, however, there may be infectious pain in the feet. In some cases, there may be no skin lesions but rather Kaposi's lymphosarcomas. These submucosal skin lesions are red or purple and are commonly seen in the mouth on the gums, hard palate, soft palate, root of the tongue, or back wall of the pharynx. In addition, half or more of KS cases may show one or more types of gastrointestinal distress. The sarcoma can also affect the lungs, spleen, heart, liver, and kidneys.

Other malignant tumors include malignant lymphomas, lymphoblastic lymphosarcomas, Hodgkin's disease, rectal squamous carcinoma, and rectal lingulate carcinoma.

In short, AIDS is a disease which may present in many systems all over the body. Some patients may primarily show irregularities of the nervous system. The main nervous disorders include inflammations of the nervous system and localized nervous degeneration caused by metabolic disorders. Commonly seen symptoms include dizziness, headache, weak limbs, epilepsy, progressive dementia, hallucinations, and localized nervous symptoms. The primary pathogens infecting the central nervous system are *Toxoplasma*, cytomegalovirus, herpes simplex virus, retrovirus, *Mycobacteria avium*, and *Pneumocystis* bacteria.

AIDS can also affect the eyes on a large scale. These symptoms usually appear in the advanced stage. The most frequent manifestations are cotton-wool patches, cytomegalovirus keratitis, conjunctivitis, Kaposi's sarcoma on the conjunctiva and eyelids, *Mycobacterium avian* choroid granulomatosis, and toxoplasmatic retinitis. These pathogens may attack any part of the eye and, in time, cause diminished vision and even blindness.

IV. The Present State of Treatment for AIDS

The current treatment of AIDS mostly consists of controlling various injuries to the body caused by AIDS, such as the control of opportunistic infections by antibiotics and other drugs. The effective drugs for AIDS are basically divided into two categories, namely antiviral preparations and immune regulators.

Antiviral preparations include AZT, ribavirin, suramin, 2-interferon, HPA-23, and glycyrrhizin. Immunopotentiators include T-peptide, isopropyl inosine, interleukin-2, lentinan, Y-interferon, and antithymosin 2-1. While immunosuppressants include cyclocytidene A and cyclophosphamide. Another approach sometimes used to rebuild normal immunity is injection of fresh thyroid cells into the body of AIDS patients.

All the above drugs have some therapeutic effect although none offer a complete cure. Unfortunately, many of these also have serious side effects. AZT is, at present, the usual drug of first choice. Inside the body, it can completely inhibit reverse transcriptase thus hindering the production of the virus' nucleoprotein. This improves the clinical symptoms and prolongs survival time. It does not, however, improve the condition of the underlying immunological disturbance. What's more, it has to be taken both indefinitely and frequently. This means not only a large expense but severe side effects as well. Examples of these side effects are inhibition of the bone marrow's hemopoiesis as well as digestive tract symptoms and nervous disorders. Because of these reasons, patients have great difficulty with this approach.

Recently in the United States, new drugs called DDC and DDI which are similar to AZT have begun to be used. DDC demonstrates antiviral activity *in vitro* and is currently being tested clinically. Continued clinical research is still required regarding its side effects.

From the above, we can see that the modern Western medical treatment of AIDS is still in its research stage and, so far, there is no completely satisfactory treatment. On the other hand, Traditional Chinese Medicine has a certain advantage with its vast experience in improving body immunity and inhibiting viral activity. What's more, when Chinese medicine is administered correctly, there are *no side effects*. At present, the treatment of AIDS with TCM has attracted much interest abroad. Some clinicians have already begun researching the treatment of AIDS with Traditional Chinese Medicine.

2

Ai Zi Bing De Bing Yin Bing Ji

AIDS, Its Etiology & Pathophysiology

I. *Zu Guo Yi Xue Dui Ai Zi Bing De Ren Shi* The Categorization of AIDS According to TCM Theory

Over thousands of years, Chinese medicine has accumulated rich experience in the treatment and prevention of disease. In modern times with the continued development of TCM, great progress has been made in the prevention and TCM treatment of infectious diseases, such as viral hepatitis, as well as of hypoimmunity, lupus erythematosus, malignant tumors, and a number of functional disorders. AIDS was first officially named in 1983. It is an infectious disease which has spread throughout the world in recent years. Because it is a new disease, there is no previous, direct research on this disease in TCM from the past. However, TCM does already possess a large body of knowledge regarding similar diseases and symptoms. Based on its clinical manifestations and the result of foreign scholars' research combining both TCM and modern medicine, AIDS can be compared to other conditions in TCM which have been well researched and delineated.

The *Su Wen: Ci Fa Lun (Simple Questions: Treatise on Needling Methods)* says:

> The five epidemic diseases are all easily caught. Whether in the old or young, their symptoms are the same.

Because AIDS also shares the characteristic of other epidemic diseases, such as its serious nature and consistent symptoms, it should be classified as an "infectious epidemic disease" or *yi bing* according to TCM. Also, since the disease is caused by viral evils invading internally during vacuity which then hide in the *xue luo* or blood network vessels and inside the *ying fen* or constructive aspect, the symptoms of this warm hot disease or *wen re bing* should also be categorized as a species of *wen yi* or "pestilence". This disease has a relatively long latent period, a sudden onset, and severe symptoms. When the *wen re xie du* or warm hot evil toxins attack outward, there may be bleeding symptoms, such as macular eruptions, nosebleed, blood in the urine, spitting blood, and blood in the stools; symptoms of stagnation and accumulation of hot toxins; or even symptoms of extreme heat causing stirring of wind. Therefore, this disease may also be classified as a *fu qi wen bing* or "hidden qi warm disease". Wang Meng-ying, a scholar in the Qing Dynasty, said:

> Hidden qi warm diseases go from inside to outside or from *li* to *biao*. They begin in the *xue fen* and extend to the *qi fen*...This is quite different from external invasion of warm evils which go from *wei* to *qi* to *ying* to *xue*.

What's more, this disease is usually accompanied by the clinical manifestations of source or *yuan qi* weakness and damage and *jing qi* or essence qi insufficiency. These include progressive emaciation, fatigue, night sweats, poor appetite, and diarrhea. In the *Jin Gui Yao Lue (Essentials from the Golden Cabinet)*, such symptoms have been recorded in the chapter on "The Theory of Vacuity Taxation (*Xu Lao*)": "Vacuous pulse, face color pale, face color white, palpitations, emaciation, inability to walk due to sore and thin skin, blurred vision, withered hair, subaxillary lymphadenopathy, night sweats, loose stools, diarrhea, cramping or distention in the lower abdomen or even diarrhea with undigested food in the stools, nocturnal emissions..." From this, it is clear that AIDS is very similar to a *xu sun* or vacuity detriment disease in TCM. In particular, *xu sun* accompanied by subaxillary lymphadenopathy is surprisingly similar to AIDS with its prolonged diarrhea due to infection of the intestinal tract and lymphadenopathy. As early as the *Nei Jing (Internal Classic)*, there was already a record of *xu lao* or vacuity taxation. In the *Su Wen: Yu Ji Zhen Zang Lun (Simple Questions: Crucial Discussion of the True Organs [as Precious as] Jade)*, there is the following description: "Big bones withered away, big flesh drooping and sunken, stuffy qi within the chest, panting for breath and not defecating, internal pain stretching to the shoulders, body feverish, flesh and muscles worn out and ragged, shoulder marrow inside vanished, movement increasingly declines." Based on its clinical manifestations similar to those above, AIDS can also be classified as a species of *xu lao* (vacuity taxation) or *wu lao xu sun* (five taxations vacuity detriment).

Usually, AIDS is accompanied by lymphadenopathy. This is categorized as *luo li* or scrofula in TCM. It is recorded in the *Ling Shu: Han Re Pian (Miraculous Pivot: Essay on Fever & Chills)*:

> Fever and chills and scrofula arise in the neck and armpit. Where does the qi that causes this come from?

> Qi Bo answered: The fever and chills of scrofula are due to toxic qi which accumulates in the vessels and is not discharged.

From this it can be seen that, in the *Nei Jing*, there is not only mention of scrofula but also the saying that it is due to toxic evils invading the inside of the body. Also, in the *Bian Zheng Lu (On the Differentiation of Patterns)* written in the Qing Dynasty, it is said:

> Scrofula is mostly caused by phlegm, but phlegm mostly arises due to depression. If there is no depression, phlegm cannot arise. And

15

without phlegm, there is no scrofula.

Based on clinical experience, AIDS may worsen due to evil toxins hidden internally and accumulation of phlegm stasis. Hence, in prolonged cases, there may be hepatomegaly and splenomegaly as well as malignant tumors. All these are categorized as *ji ju* (accumulations and gatherings) and *zheng jia* (concretions and conglomerations), *e he* (malignant nodules), and *shi rong* (now usually identified as cervical cancer with cachexia but originally meaning loss of flourishing [due to tumor]). The *Zhu Bing Yuan Hou Lun (Treatise on the Origin & Symptoms of Disease)* says:

> These diseases are caused by irregular cold or warm (foods) further causing vacuity and weakness of the viscera and bowels *qi* plus undigested food. These gather and knot together internally thus giving rise to masses. That which cannot be moved is a tumor.

The prolonged vacuity detriment or *xu sun* of AIDS may lead to the occurrence of *zheng jia* or concretions and conglomerations. The *Wai Sheng Bao Jian (The Precious Mirror of Hygiene)* says:

> If the spleen and stomach are vacuous and weak or food and drink are irregular, or if one eats excessive cold or hot food, (the spleen and stomach) may not be able to transform food. Hence accumulation, stagnation, gathering, and knotting cause lumps.

Though there may be many causes, *zheng jia ji ju* or abdominal masses in AIDS are usually due to insufficiency of righteous qi. Zhang Jie-gu said:

> Strong people do not have stagnations/accumulations. Weak (literally vacuous) people have these.

The name *shi rong* (loss of flourishing [due to tumor]) was first recorded in the *Wai Ke Zheng Zong: Shi Rong Bing (Orthodox Manual of External Disease: Loss of Flourishing Disease)*. The lymphadenopathy and malignant tumors in AIDS are usually similar to this disease. This is vividly described in the *Yong Ke Chuan Xin De Ji (A Collection of Clinical Experiences in the Treatment of Ulcers)*: "Just as trees lose their verdure, their branches and bark becoming dry and thin, hence the name consumption."

If the evil toxins of AIDS invade upwards to the brain, there may be convulsions or dementia which are similar to the symptoms of *dian xian* or epilepsy in TCM. It is said in the *Gu Ling Yi Jian (Ancient Ode of the Mirror of Medicine)*, "It attacks with sudden collapse, mouth and eyes deviated, convulsions, stiff neck and back, and drooling." Its onset is discussed in the *Dan Xi Xin Fa ([Zhu] Dan-Xi's Essential Methods)*:

> The depressive type is categorized as yin, while the manic type is categorized as yang. Both are caused primarily by phlegm knotting in the chest.

Hence it can be seen that phlegm evil is the main cause of this condition. This is shown even more clearly in the *Yi Xue Gang Mu (A Detailed Outline of Medical Theory)*, "Epilepsy is caused by the upward counterflow of phlegm evil." Over time, AIDS patients tend to show exhaustion of viscera and bowels function and repeated invasion by external evils which may quickly worsen the case leading to a serious situation where there is a preponderance of evil qi and a waning of the righteous. This then results in the coming apart of yin and yang (with yang flushing upward).

II. *Ai Zi Bing De Bing Yin/Bing Ji* Etiology & Pathophysiology of AIDS

Traditional Chinese Medicine believes that the human body is an organic whole. Health and normal function are maintained by a relative balance between the organs and tissues as well as between the human body and the external environment. The factors which can cause imbalance are many. AIDS may present a variety of clinical manifestations, but all its *bing yin* or causative factors are included under *nei yin* (internal causes), *wai yin* (external causes), and *bu nei bu wai yin* (neither internal nor external causes). Its external causes are mainly evil toxins and invasion by pestilential qi. Its internal causes are mainly vacuity of qi and blood, viscera and bowels. External evils usually invade the human body when the inside is vacuous. In other words, they attack when there is already an internal imbalance. Phlegm dampness and blood stasis are two pathogenic products which arise due to imbalance in the function of the viscera and bowels, qi and blood in AIDS. These pathogenic factors may result in the formation of carbuncles, nodulations, scrofula, and malignant tumors in AIDS patients. Since this disease is a systemic disease effecting the entire body, more attention should be paid to its internal causative factors.

A. *Yi Xie Gan Ran*
Infection by Pestilential Evils

Epidemic evils are especially strong infectious pathogens which cause diseases characterized by sudden and rapid onset with severe and consistent symptoms, strong infectiousness, and extreme communicability. Wu You-ke of the Ming Dynasty referred to these factor as *li qi* or pestilential qi. In his book, the *Wen Yi Lun (Treatise on Warm Diseases)*, he pointed out that, "Warm epidemics are not caused by wind, cold, summer heat, or dampness but by a strange sort of qi affecting the space between heaven and earth." In fact, this pestilential qi is a special kind of pathogen. According to modern medicine, AIDS is caused by HIV infection. This is called a pestilential evil in TCM. The *Su Wen (Simple Questions)* says:

> Essence is the root of the body. Therefore, when essence is treasured, there are no warm diseases in the spring.

Hence it can be seen that treasuring or storing kidney essence is a key point in the prevention of warm hot diseases. Hua Tuo, in his *Zhong Zang Jing (Classic of the Central Treasury)*, said, "If one's qi and blood are waning and weak and one's viscera and bowels are vacuous, they may be affected by evil qi which can thus cause disease..." Therefore, pestilential evils mostly afflict those whose body's viscera and bowels source qi is vacuous and damaged.

The AIDS virus usually spreads through the interpersonal exchange of body fluids, such as sperm or blood. Its infection is usually due to excessive or abnormal sex which consumes and injures true yang. This results in an vacuity of righteous (qi) due to the kidneys not treasuring essence, and viral evils may invade via the five fluids and other body fluids coincidental to an vacuous condition. Thus pestilential evils take advantage of a body which is vacuous.

According to TCM theory, there also exists the possibility of asymptomatic infection by pestilential toxins which then show symptoms when the body's righteous qi later becomes deficient and vacuous. Pestilential toxic evils can also spread via the blood. In Chinese medicine, this is referred to as *wu xue* or "polluted blood". This includes various blood products and even the spread from the mother's body to the fetus. After invading the body, viral evils lie hidden in the *xue luo* or blood network vessels and house themselves internally within the *ying* or constructive aspect. Thus this disease occurs.

B. *Zang Fu Qi Xue Xu Sun*
Vacuity & Damage of the Viscera and Bowels, Qi & Blood

Vacuity and fullness are two aspects in the struggle between the body's resistance to disease and disease evils. Vacuity refers to insufficiency of righteous qi, decrease of the body's resistance to disease, and hypofunction of physiological activities. The onset of AIDS is usually due to a combination of vacuity and detriment (*xu sun*) of the qi and blood and viral evils taking advantage of this vacuity. As stated in the *Nei Jing*, "If evil has the chance to collect, one's qi must be vacuous." Xu Chun-pu said,

> If a person habitually protects and enriches their qi and values their
> essence and blood, evil cannot invade. But if a man indulges/releases
> his desire excessively and wantonly and is not conscious and aware,

blood and essence will be consumed inside and evil qi will take advantage.

The onset of AIDS is almost always like this. Liu Wan-su said, "Vacuity detriment diseases are due to cold and hot *yin* or disease causing factors plus vacuity." Zhang Jing-yue also said, "A person whose spleen and stomach are insufficient, vacuous, weak, and not balanced usually have *ji ju* or gathering and accumulation diseases." When the body is vacuous and weak and viscera and bowels function is imbalanced, sensitivity to viral evils increases and the stability of the internal environment is destroyed. Because disease resistance is weak, external evils are likely to invade. Whether there is an occurrence of disease after viral evils have invaded the body does not depend solely on the presence of viral evils but also on the body's resistance. If the body's resistance is strong enough, the infected individual will remain an asymptomatic carrier of HIV.

According to TCM, the kidneys store essence and control growth and reproduction. They also control the five kinds of body fluids and thus are the or water organ. Both prenatal and postnatal essence are stored in the kidneys. Therefore, they are called the prenatal root. When the source yin and source yang of the kidneys is vacuous and damaged, it may cause vacuity and detriment in the function of the other viscera and bowels. This allows disease to arise in the body. According to modern medical theory, vacuity and detriment of the viscera and bowels usually present as hypoimmunity and especially hypofunction of both cellular and humoral immunity. When the body loses its immunity, diseases occur. In TCM, immune function is a combination of qi gathered in the center and source qi rooted in the kidneys. This is transported all over the body through the triple burner activating and promoting the functional activities of all the viscera and bowels. Vacuity and detriment of the viscera and bowels in AIDS mainly affects three organs—the lungs, spleen, and kidneys. Among these, kidney yin and yang, *i.e.*, source yin and yang, regulate the yin and yang of the entire body. Therefore, vacuity and detriment or *xu sun* of kidney yin and/or yang are main causative factors.

C. *Qing Zhi Suo Shang*
Injury Due to Emotions

Human emotions include joy, anger, melancholy, worry, grief, fear, and fright. If there is prolonged mental/emotional stress or sudden mental/emotional trauma, these go beyond their normal functional regulation causing disorder in the flow·of qi and abnormal functioning of the viscera and bowels, yin and yang, qi and blood. Most AIDS patients are homosexuals and are likely to express avoidance psychology toward their friends, colleagues, employers, and others. Therefore, they often experience attitudinal changes and are sometimes nervous, worried, or depressed. To make matters worse, when so affected, they tend to look increasingly for excessive stimulation through smoking, alcohol, or other activities leading to an even worse mental and physical state. All this may cause a series of pathological changes, such as "melancholy damaging the spleen" or "anger damaging the liver", and further lead to deficiency and vacuity of the viscera and bowels, qi and blood as well as imbalance of the qi mechanism. On hearing the diagnosis of AIDS, a patient may also experience a series of abnormal mental/emotional changes. They may be shocked, angry, depressed, or worried, some even fainting in sudden fright. These severe mental changes may worsen the situation, thus leading to deterioration.

Mental disorders usually cause disorder of the qi thus manifesting diseases caused by qi disorder. In the course of AIDS, patients' cases are often complicated by the pathological change of liver qi stagnation evidenced by worry or depression. If the liver loses its normal function of maintaining the free flow of qi, this results in stagnation of qi. Prolonged stagnation of qi may affect the blood causing blood stasis which may further affect the five viscera. Therefore, in advanced AIDS, one typically encounters a number of pathological changes caused by stagnant qi and blood stasis.

D. *Fang Lao Guo Du*
Excessive Sexual Taxation

The kidneys store the essence and control treasuring and banking. When kidney essence is sufficient, the human is able to maintain their normal physiological functions. Before the onset of AIDS, patients often have experienced excessive or abnormal sex which may have exhausted their essence and fluids and scattered their true qi. When the kidneys fail to store essence, the viscera and bowels become deficient and damaged. Viral evils may take advantage of this vacuity, thus resulting in the onset of this disease.

E. *Qi Zhi Xue Yu*
Qi Stagnation & Blood Stasis

Qi is the basic material constituent in the maintenance of the life, activity, and strength of the human body. Qi and blood are closely related. Qi can produce blood and promote its movement. In other words, the transportation and movement of blood and fluids relies on the movement of qi. Vacuity of qi results in vacuity of blood, and stagnation of qi in blood stasis. Normally, qi is able to move up, down, in, and out and move all over the entire body. But due to the various mental changes accompanying AIDS discussed above, such as worry and depression, there may be such pathological changes as the stagnation and binding of liver qi. This causes the pathological change of the qi mechanism not being free and unimpeded. Qi stagnation results in the blood not being free and unimpeded, and slow blood circulation eventually leads to blood stasis. In addition, since, the viscera and bowels, qi and blood of AIDS patients are deficient and vacuous, vacuous qi fails to promote the normal circulation of blood and fluids which also leads to blood stasis. As stated in the *Jing Yue Quan Shu ([Zhang] Jing-yue's Complete Writings)*:

> Peoples' qi and blood flow like a stream. If the current is sufficient, it flows smoothly. But if the current is insufficient, the flow is diminished. If qi and blood are not vacuous, there is no stagnation.

Without vacuity, there is no stagnation.

Also, in the *Du Yi Sui Bi: Cheng Zhi Sheng Hua Lun (Medical Notes: Treatise on Formation & Transformation)*, it is clearly stated that, "If vacuous qi is insufficient to promote blood circulation, this will surely result in blood stasis." In the case of AIDS, all the viscera and bowels, qi and blood are deficient and weak; so blood stasis is very likely. The *Bu Ji* says, "All consumptive diseases are accompanied by blood stasis," and, "With consumption, the patient becomes emaciated, and because of blood stasis internally, there may be flaky, dry skin externally." After the accumulation of static blood, the blood not only loses its normal nourishing function but, in turn, affects the circulation and transportation of blood and fluids of the entire body.If prolonged qi stagnation and blood stasis are not scattered, they may give rise internally to *zheng jia ji ju* or abdominal masses in the viscera.

F. *Tan Shi Ning Zhi*
Phlegm Dampness Congelation & Stagnation

Phlegm rheum are species of pathological products in the human body due to a variety of pathogenic factors. After the formation of phlegm or rheum it can affect the viscera and bowels directly or indirectly, thus causing disease. The three organs whose function controls the normal regulation of water fluids are the lungs, spleen, and kidneys. The lungs control dispersing and descending. They course and balance the water passageways and distribute fluids and humors. The spleen controls transportation and transformation of water fluids. The kidneys control the evaporation of water fluids and the triple burner is the pathway through which water fluids flow freely and are balanced. When viscera dn bowel function is deficient and damaged, qi and blood circulation is impeded. This affects the functions of the lungs, spleen, and kidneys *vis à vis* the dispersion and expulsion of water fluids, thus causing accumulation of water dampness. Further accumulation of dampness congeals into phlegm. In the *Dan Xi Xin Fa*, there is the saying, "The pathological product, phlegm, rises and falls with the qi and goes to all places."

After the formation of phlegm rheum, it can present various manifestations in different locations. If phlegm stagnates in the lungs, there is typically cough and asthma with mucous. If phlegm knots in the channels and network vessels, between the sinews and the bones, under the skin, or within the flesh, there may be phlegm nodulation and scrofula, numb limbs, or hemiplegia. If phlegm turbidity attacks upwards to the head, there may be dizziness and vertigo. In the later stages of AIDS, phlegm may block the heart and befuddle the heart orifices. In this case, patients usually experience unconsciousness, dementia, or epilepsy. Phlegm turbidity and blood stasis may bind together and may combine with evil toxins. This blocks the body internally and may give rise to scrofula and other, malignant tumors.

III. Recapitulation of Etiology & Pathophysiology

More than 2,000 years ago, Traditional Chinese Medicine already believed that the viscera and bowels and channels and network vessels of the human body maintain a relative balance with the outer environment. Under normal circumstances, the viscera and bowels and channels and network vessels also maintain a relative balance in physiological activities between the qi and blood and yin and yang. In other words, "When yin is stabilized and yang well conserved, the spirit is harmonious." When the human body is affected by some pathogenic factor, the viscera and bowels and channels and network vessels function abnormally and this relative balance between qi and blood and yin and yang is destroyed. Hence the occurrence of disease and pathological change.

TCM believes these physiological activities and pathological changes are all the manifestation of righteous and evil qi. That is, though AIDS may have different causes and manifestations, its course and symptoms are all related to either the righteous qi of the body or the evil qi. If the viscera and bowels function normally, there is sufficient righteous qi, sufficient blood, and stable defensive qi. Evil qi cannot invade and disease does not occur. As stated in the *Su Wen: Ci Fa Lun,* "Evil cannot invade from without if righteous qi defends the body from within." However, if righteous qi becomes vacuous and defensive qi is too weak to resist the invasion of evils, viral evils may invade causing imbalance of yin and yang and further vacuity in the function of the channels and network vessels and hence the occurrence of disease. In the *Su Wen: Wen Re Lun (Simple Questions: Treatise on Warmth & Heat),* it is said, "Where evil qi invades, defensive qi must be weak." It is also stated in the *Ling Shu,* "Cold or heat, wind or rain, if there is no deficiency of the righteous, evil cannot affect the body." From the clinical point of view, it has been proven that all HIV patients do not necessarily demonstrate symptoms of disease but only those who lack the antiviral antigen. Therefore, it is quite clear that whether one develops AIDS mainly depends on the state of the body resistance. That is, the deficiency of righteous qi is the internal breeding ground of AIDS.

While emphasizing the function of the righteous in the occurrence of AIDS, we do not exclude the function of the disease evils. It should be pointed out that, under some circumstances, external evils may be the main cause. For instance, it should not be overlooked that there are many AIDS cases resulting from injection, blood transfusion, the use of contaminated blood products, or infection from pregnant mother to infant. Therefore, it has also been pointed out in the *Nei Jing* that we should "avoid toxic qi" so as to prevent infection.

The relationship between righteous qi and evil determines not only the occurrence of AIDS but also its development and prognosis. Generally speaking, during increase of righteous qi due to recovery of viscera and bowel function, qi and blood, the case may stabilize or improve. Similarly, if evil qi increases, righteous qi may gradually decrease, resulting in the body's inability to resist evil factors. As this goes on, the case worsens rapidly or additional infection by external evils prove fatal.

Also, it should not be overlooked that there is a close relationship between the mental state and the occurrence of this disease. Though AIDS virus carriers may show no symptoms, their psychological condition is often under great strain. Such mental/emotional changes often cause abnormal viscera and bowel function with concomitant vacuity of righteous qi. This may result in the rapid development of ARC or further worsen the case. As stated in the *Su Wen*, "Living peacefully with no desire for fame or gain and keeping the source qi within prevents the body from being infected by disease." Therefore, normal mental/emotional activities enhance the righteous qi, reducing or preventing the occurrence and development of AIDS.

Traditional Chinese Medicine believes that the pathophysiology of AIDS is mainly comprised of two broad categories of pathological changes. One category is comprised of changes encountered in the course of involvement of external evils. These pathological changes are none other than the manifestation of pathological functioning of the viscera and bowels as governed by the triple burner. These changes are due to the abnormal function of the defensive qi and constructive and blood phases in turn caused by infection by epidemic toxins. The other broad category is comprised of those pathological changes manifesting in the course of internal disorders. This refers to those pathological changes due to deficiency and vacuity of the viscera and bowels, qi and blood, and yin and yang or the transformation of the mixture of fullness and vacuity in advanced stages.

Evil qi invades the body when righteous qi is weak and the defensive qi is unconsolidated or *bu gu*. This may result in "epidemic warm evils invading the upper" portion of the body or the lungs first. This usually presents with symptoms of "the lungs being affected by evil", such as fever, fear of draft, cough, and a superficial pulse. There may also be symptoms of heat in the *yang ming* or qi phase due to direct invasion of the *qi fen* by epidemic evils. If warm evils and hot toxins accumulate internally, they may block the flow of qi thus causing dampness. If damp heat accumulates in the middle burner or *zhong jiao*, there will be thrush, stomachache, erosion or sores in the mouth, and a dry, powdery tongue coating. If pestilential evil accumulates in the blood or constructive phases, heat may erupt from the skin and flesh causing hemorrhage or skin rashes.

Excessive sex may exhaust source yin. Therefore, kidney disorders are the main internal disease. Also, there is a close relationship between the viscera and bowels and the kidneys. Kidney yin and yang are the basis of body fluids (yin) and yang qi. For this reason, disorders of the kidneys may not only cause imbalance in their own yin and yang but also affect other organs as well. That is why this disease is often accompanied by vacuity of many of the viscera and bowels as well as of yin and yang and qi and blood.

According to an analysis of clinical research, the affected organs are mainly the spleen, lungs, and kidneys with vacuity of yin or yang of any of these three viscera. Different viscus disorders present different signs and symptoms. If kidney essence is insufficient, there may be internal vacuity of yin with such symptoms of kidney yin vacuity as night sweats, fever, emaciation, etc. Vacuity of kidney yin may also affect the lungs. This is a disorder of the child affecting the mother according to "mother-child theory". This may cause vacuous fire flaring upward burning lung fluids with such symptoms of injury of both lung qi and lung yin as dry cough with little mucous, slight fever with night or spontaneous sweats, shortness of breath, feeble voice, fatigue, etc. If the spleen and blood are deficient and vacuous, the postnatal root may become insufficient. When central qi is weak, it cannot transport nutrient essence. This results in weak limbs and emaciation. If the spleen loses its function of transportation and transformation, dampness cannot be dissolved properly. Hence loose stools and diarrhea. If this lasts, there will be signs of vacuity of both spleen and kidneys, such as fear of cold, cold limbs, and prolonged diarrhea.

To make matters worse, the above pathological changes often affect each other between themselves which may complicate and worsen the case. Pestilential evils are most likely to injure the righteous qi. This not only worsens injury to the viscera and bowel deterioration. Finally the patient may present fatal signs of exhaustion of both kidney yin and yang, viscera and bowels, and qi and blood, such as cachexia, bone atrophy, and declining vitality. Therefore, this disease is quite different from simple vacuity taxation (*xu lao, i.e.,* consumption) or viscera and bowel vacuity. Here, the vacuity of the viscera and bowels and qi and blood are both an internal factor allowing for evil invasion and the occurrence of the disease *and* the result of the pathological changes due to invasion by those evils. In turn, this vacuity causes the toxic evils to further invade and accumulate, thus forming a vicious cycle.

Viscera and bowel, qi and blood vacuity and abnormal function often result in the pathogenesis of phlegm rheum and blood stasis. When the qi is too weak to promote movement, blood becomes static and accumulates inside leading to hepatomegaly and splenomegaly or tumors, abdominal lumps, and masses. If blood stasis binds and accumulates with phlegm, there will be scrofula and other, malignant tumors. When phlegm disturbs the mind, there will be dementia or aphasia. And if phlegm fire disturbs upward, there will be epilepsy, mania, or delirium which may further worsen the case. Meanwhile, due to insufficiency of righteous qi, the viscera and bowels and qi and blood may become even emptier and the defensive qi further unconsolidated. In the course of disease, further infection by external evils at this stage may often worsen the case leading to the coming apart of yin and yang.

Consumption or vacuity taxation and infection by toxic evils are, therefore, seen as the key disease causing factors. Therefore, in the treatment of this disease, the etiology should be clearly examined and the main symptoms determined. Also, the relationship between the righteous and evil qi should be differentiated so as to prevent the further development of this disease.

3

Ai Zi Bing De Zhi Liao Yuan Ze

Therapeutic Principles In the Treatment of AIDS

The hallmarks of TCM theory are its holistic view of the various parts of the body as an organic whole and its selection of treatment based on a discrimination of patterns or *bian zheng*. These two principles should be the basis of the TCM treatment of AIDS. Only by treating insightfully according to the different situations can a good result be obtained and the goal of treatment be achieved. The administration of each and every treatment, prescription, and herbal medicinal should be guided by these principles. AIDS is a systemic disorder caused by a number of disease causes affecting a number of organs and systems. Based on its various different symptoms, we can say that its pathological changes are quite complicated and its course may vary. In other words, the situation differs in different individuals and at various stages in the course of this disease. Therefore, one should abide by the selection of treatment on the basis of pattern discrimination, aiming at the root cause, discriminating acute from chronic and primary from secondary. This means that one should support the righteous and eliminate evil according to the fluctuations in emptiness and fullness in the struggle between righteous and evil. In this way, treatment takes into account the whole body and may postpone the continued development of AIDS. Thus the goal of treatment is obtained.

I. *Bian Bing Yu Bian Zheng* Disease Discrimination/Pattern Discrimination

TCM treatment methodology is characterized by *bian zheng lun zhi* or the selection of treatment on the basis of a discrimination of patterns. However, TCM also administers treatment based on *bian bing lun zhi*. This is treatment based on the *bing* or disease. The *zheng* or pattern is the total *gestalt* of the individual patient as ascertained by the 4 diagnoses (*si zhen*) and analyzed according to the 8 principles (*ba gang*). It includes all an individual patient's signs and symptoms besides those which are strictly pathognomic of their disease. *Bing* or disease refers to both named disease categories and individual signs and symptoms. For instance, AIDS is a *bing* and so are cough, dizziness, and lymphadenopathy. Treatment based on disease discrimination is directed at either the patient's signs and symptoms or at the particular idiosyncracies of an individual disease.

The manifestations of AIDS are due not only to the quality and quantity of the HIV pathogen but also to individual differences in particular patients. Therefore, in the course of this disease, clinical symptoms vary from person to person. This is why the treatment of AIDS should be based on both disease discrimination (*bian bing*) and pattern discrimination (*bian zheng*). By basing treatment on an overall assessment of the individual patient or a *bian zheng* diagnosis, one can take into account and address the individual differences in various patients who may all be suffering from the same disease. This is the meaning of the saying,

> *Yi bing, tong zhi; Tong bing, yi zhi.*
>
> One disease, different treatments;
> Different diseases, one treatment.

That is not to say, however, that treatment should not also be based on modern clinical test results. Such methods of modern *bian bing* diagnosis help establish a clearer diagnostic picture and compensate for some of the shortcomings of TCM diagnosis. Thus one should also insightfully employ treatment methods based not only on pattern discrimination but also on disease discrimination as well, remembering that a *bing* may refer to either a disease as a whole or an individual symptom. For example, one may add some antiviral herbs to improve immunity or some anti-opportunistic infection or tumor-inhibiting herbs based on a *bian bing* understanding of the disease in order to achieve a better overall effect. In short, in clinical practice it is extremely important to analyze the patient's condition as completely as possible using both *bian bing* and *bian zheng*.

II. *Zhi Biao Yu Zhi Ben*
Treating the Branch/Treating the Root

Branch and root are two interdependent concepts in TCM which describe the primary and secondary aspects in the course of a disease. Primary and secondary symptoms as well as acute and chronic conditions may be categorized according to differences between internal and external, righteous and evil, cause and manifestation, and the sequence of a disease's progression. Based on this discrimination, one may decide whether to treat the root first and then the branch, the branch first and then the root, or root and branch simultaneously. As stated in the *Su Wen (Simple Questions)*:

> Doctors who know root and branch always treat correctly. Those who do not understand these often fail to cure disease.

Thus the importance of discriminating root and branch in the erection of a treatment plan can be seen.

Because AIDS usually manifests clinically as a deficiency and emptiness of righteous qi and consequent severe immune deficiency, treatment of the root by supporting the righteous often is given precedence. Thus, by treating the root, the branch is treated automatically. This is known as treating the root first in more chronic conditions. As stated in the *Nei Jing*, "To treat disease, one must surely seek the root."

Although the etiology of AIDS is very complicated, its clinical manifestations usually demonstrate a clear difference between root and branch. For instance, AIDS is usually accompanied by many kinds of fatal opportunistic infections. If these are not well controlled but one only supports the righteous qi, the case will quickly worsen and often with fatal consequences. This is a good example of a branch symptom becoming the most important aspect of the disease. Here, the secondary symptoms are more urgent than the primary one; so they should be treated first. After the infections have been controlled and the secondary symptoms relieved, the primary ones should be treated so as to improve the state of deficiency detriment of the righteous qi. This is known as treating the branch first in acute situations.

However, if both the branch and root diseases or symptoms are urgent, they should be treated simultaneously. For example, in the advanced stage of AIDS, there may be phlegm nodulations or concretions and conglomerations, accumulations and gatherings due to enlargement of the liver and/or spleen and other, malignant tumors which result in tumor obstruction, tumor pressure, tumor transmission, and tumor spreading which damage the internal organs. Meanwhile, the functions of the viscera and bowels and qi and blood are very weak. In this case, only treating either root or branch is not sufficient. Both should be treated simultaneously. Thus, the rule of treating both the root and branch together should be applied. Only by using both the eliminating and the supplementing method at the same time can this disease be cured. In other words, treatment should be based on reinforcing the righteous as the root as well as combatting the tumor in order to relieve the symptoms or the branch.

The relationship between root and branch is complex. Distinctions between primary and secondary concerns typically alternate as the disease develops. Therefore, one must be able to change the treatment plan flexibly as the disease changes and transforms. From the above examples, it is clear that treatment principles based on a discrimination of root and branch should not only be applied according to the tenets of TCM theory but also with a sense of adaptability. When employed in clinical practice, the relationships between root and branch, primary and secondary, cause and result, mild and severe, and chronic and acute should always be taken into account. In acute cases, treat the branch or urgent symptoms. In chronic cases, treat the root or both the root and branch together to cure the root cause. These are the basic principles of treating AIDS according to a discrimination of root and branch.

III. *Fu Zheng Yu Qu Xie*
Supporting the Righteous/
Eliminating the Evil

Supporting the righteous means to support the righteous qi, strengthen the body's resistance, and improve immune function. Eliminating evil means to eliminate, inhibit, and expel the disease causes, such as the AIDS virus.

The onset of AIDS is mostly due to deficiency detriment of the viscera and bowels. Therefore, supporting the righteous should be the main treatment. In other words, one should, depending upon the symptoms of vacuity and detriment of yin and yang, qi and blood, viscera and bowels, apply various kinds of supplementing methods, such as boosting the qi, supplementing the blood, nourishing yin, and assisting yang. Thus one supports the righteous and supplements emptiness, builds resistance and cures insufficiency.

From the point of view of immunity, the body's normal immunity is supposed to maintain the relative balance between the internal and external environments, improve resistance, fight the invasion of pathogens, and provide immune surveillance. When there is a viral infection, immunity is affected, causing immune deficiency. This affects source yin and yang and hence the occurrence of disease. In TCM, treatment based on pattern discrimination is designed to regulate yin and yang, qi and blood, and the function of the viscera and bowels and channels and network vessels. Thus righteous qi is supported, resistance is strengthened, evil pathogens are eliminated, and the goal of recovery is achieved.

In addition, it should be noted that supporting the righteous creates the necessary conditions for eliminating evil, while eliminating evil preserves the righteous. These two principles should be considered in the clinic when determining which, *i.e.*, righteous or evil, is more urgently in need of treatment. If attention is paid only to eliminating evil, righteous qi may be negatively affected and so resistance may be weakened. On the other hand, if attention is paid only to supporting the righteous by using only supplementing but no eliminating medicinals, the virus may relapse, further injuring the body. Therefore, in clinical practice, treatment should be directed at the righteous qi to strengthen resistance and at the disease evils in order to disperse and eliminate viral evils from the body.

Patients in the initial stage usually suffer from emptiness of the righteous. This results in the pestilential evil's ability to invade internally. In this stage, treatment should both support the righteous and eliminate evil. Those in the middle stage are usually accompanied by phlegm turbidity. If the righteous qi is strong enough to stand the attack, treatment may consist of clearing heat and resolving toxins, transforming phlegm, softening the hard, and scattering nodulation. Some herbs to support the righteous should be added to aid in eliminating disease evils. In the advanced stage, the prolonged presence of phlegm results in great emptiness of righteous qi. This causes malignant nodules and tumors. Therefore, in this stage, treatment should mainly aim at supporting the righteous with some evil-eliminating herbs as adjuvants. When the body's constitutional condition has improved, one may apply evil-eliminating herbs, thus attacking and supplementing simultaneously.

In the treatment of AIDS, one must use both the TCM principles or methods of supporting the righteous and eliminating evil. Supporting the righteous herbs usually have the function of improving the body's immunity. While eliminating evil herbs inhibit abnormal immune reactions. For example, herbs for clearing heat and resolving toxins, quickening the blood and transforming stasis, and softening the hard and scattering nodulation usually inhibit abnormal immune reaction and viral activity. They also tend to possess anti-inflammatory and anti-allergic functions. In short, by supporting the righteous and eliminating evil, *i.e.,* "supplementing insufficiency and draining excess", a general recovery may be obtained.

IV. *Chang Yong Zhi Fa* Commonly Used Treatment Methods

All the treatments herein are based on diagnosis by pattern discrimination or *bian zheng*. Only when the treatment methods (*e.g.,* clearing heat, supplementing the spleen, etc.) have been decided can they direct clinical practice and the choice of corresponding prescriptions to control the development and remission of the disease. In other words, if the *bian zheng* diagnosis identifies a pattern of spleen emptiness and an accumulation of dampness, the TCM treatment principles or methods should be to supplement the spleen and eliminate dampness. Based on this selection of treatment methods, one next chooses an appropriate formula or prescription from those categorized as supplementing the spleen and eliminating dampness.

TCM is rich in treatment methods. There are 8 basic treatment strategies, namely diaphoresis, emesis, purgation, harmonization, warming, clearing, elimination, and supplementation. These are the basis for deciding upon prescriptions. This is called "deciding prescriptions according to treatment methods." Therefore, choosing the correct treatment strategy is very important in chosing correct treatment and thus the outcome of this disease.

In TCM, there are basically two primary therapeutic approaches to AIDS. These are supporting the righteous and eliminating evil. Supporting the righteous means to strengthen the body's resistance and cultivate the root as well as to improve immunity. It also includes the treatment methods of supplementing the kidneys, spleen, and lungs. Eliminating evil means to eliminate the AIDS virus or to expel and eliminate disease evils. Practically, this means clearing heat and resolving toxins, quickening the blood and transforming stasis, and softening the hard and scattering nodulation.

A. *Fu Zheng Pei Ben*
Supporting the Righteous & Cultivating the Root

It is stated in the *Ling Shu (Miraculous Pivot)*, "Emptiness should be supplemented and fullness should be drained." Also, in the *Su Wen: Yin Yang Ying Xiang Da Lun (Simple Questions: Great Treatise on Yin & Yang)*, it is said:

> If the body is insufficient, warm with qi. If the *jing* essence is insufficient, supplement with *wei* or flavor.

Supporting and aiding the righteous qi of the body brings the body's internal environment into equilibrium with the external environment. Supporting the righteous and cultivating the root is indicated in the case of vacuity detriment of the righteous qi. For this, use supplementing and boosting prescriptions to balance and regulate the function of the viscera and bowels, qi and blood, channels and connecting vessels. Xu Zhi-cai's saying, "Supplementation is appropriate to get rid of weakness", simply summarizes this idea.

In the course of treating AIDS, the main point is to balance and supplement the lungs, spleen, and kidneys and to improve insufficiencies of qi and blood, yin and yang. It has been proven by modern Western medicine that many supplementing and boosting Chinese herbs can improve nonspecific immunity and normalize various abnormal physiological states. In clinical practice, supplementing herbs which can improve immunity include: Radix Panacis Ginseng (*Ren Shen*), Radix Astragali Membranacei (*Huang Qi*), Radix Codonopsis Pilosulae (*Dang Shen*), Rhizoma Atractylodis Macrocephalae (*Bai Zhu*), Radix Glycyrrhizae (*Gan Cao*), Prepared Radix Rehmanniae (*Shu Di*), Radix Angelicae Sinensis (*Dang Gui*), etc. Radix Astragali Membranacei (*Huang Qi*), Radix Codonopsis Pilosulae (*Dang Shen*), and Fructicatio Ganodermae Lucidae (*Ling Zhi*) can increase the production of lymphocytes and erythrocytes as well as immunoglobulin (IgA & IgG). Tuber Asparagi Cochinensis (*Tian Men Dong*), Tuber Ophiopogonis Japonicae (*Mai Men Dong*), Rhizoma Atractylodis Macrocephalae (*Bai Zhu*), Sclerotium Poriae Cocos (*Fu Ling*), Bulbus Lilii (*Bai He*), Semen Coicis Lachryma-jobi (*Yi Ren*), Radix Disocoreae Oppositae (*Shan Yao*), Radix Albus Paeoniae Lactiflorae (*Bai Shao*), Semen Germinatus Glycinis (*Dou Juan*), Semen Dolichoris Lablab (*Bian Dou*), and mushrooms can stimulate immunity, adjust hormone levels, and activate the function of certain enzymes. Fructus Mori Albi (*Sang Shen*), Ramulus Loranthi Seu Visci (*Sang Ji Sheng*), Cortex Radicis Acanthopanacis (*Wu Jia Pi*), Rhizoma Polygonati (*Huang Jing*), and other herbs containing polysaccharides, such as Shiitake mushrooms, Fructificatio Ganodermae Lucidae (*Ling Zhi*), Sclerotium Poriae Cocos (*Fu Ling*), and Sclerotium Polypori Umbellati (*Zhu Ling*), can increase T-lymphocyte blastogenesis. Radix Panacis Ginseng (*Ren Shen*) can increase immunity and has many other regulating functions as well. Other Chinese herbs, such as monkey-headed mushroom (*Hou Tou Gu*), not only increase immunity but also inhibit tumor cells.

Vacuity and detriment of the various viscera and bowels are not all the same. Therefore, supplementing and boosting methods are likewise not all the same. As stated in the *Nan Jing: Shi Si Nan (The Classic of Difficulties: 14th Difficulty)*:

> If the lungs are injured, boost the qi. If the heart is injured, balance the *ying* and *wei*. If the spleen is injured, balance eating and drinking and adjust cold and warm (foods). If the liver is injured, strike the retarded. If the kidneys are injured, boost the essence.

AIDS usually manifests deficiency and emptiness of lung, spleen, and kidney function and decline of disease resistance. Therefore, treatment should mainly be to support the righteous which means mostly to supplement these three organs. However, because the kidneys are the prenatal root and the dwelling of true yin and yang and because the spleen is the postnatal root and origin of the arisal and transformation of qi and blood, in the treatment of AIDS, supplementation of the kidneys and spleen are the key to supplementing and boosting. *The Analysis of Weakness* records:

> In the treatment of emptiness, three organs are the basis—the lungs, spleen, and kidneys. The lungs are the highest of the five organs. The spleen is the mother of the flesh. And the kidneys are the root of life. Therefore, supplementing the lungs, spleen, and kidneys includes almost all methods of treating insufficiency.

1. *Bu Pi*
Supplementing the Spleen

In the human body, emptiness and weakness of the righteous qi may have many causes. However, of these, damage and injury of the spleen and stomach are the single most common. As Li Dong-yuan said, "Injury of the spleen and stomach results in many diseases." If viral evils invade the body internally, this usually and easily damages and injures spleen qi. This then leads to emptiness and weakness of righteous qi and a decline in disease resistance. Therefore, the signs and symptoms of spleen emptiness are commonly encountered in AIDS. When such signs and symptoms are encountered, herbal medicinals should be used to supplement the qi and strengthen the spleen, thus aiding the growth of bodily resistance. For instance, *Sheng Ling Bai Zhu San* and *Xiang Sha Liu Jun Zi Tang* are representative formulas for strengthening the spleen and thus improving the body's resistance. In recent years, animal experiments have proven that herbs which strengthen the spleen stimulate phagocytosis within the reticuloendothelial system. Therefore, herbs which supplement spleen qi most definitely can strengthen resistance and improve immunity.

In clinical practice, herbs which strengthen the spleen and boost the qi include: Rhizoma Atractylodis Macrocephalae (*Bai Zhu*), Sclerotium Poriae Cocos (*Fu Ling*), Pericarpium Citri Reticulatae (*Chen Pi*), Radix Codonopsis Pilosulae (*Dang Shen*), Radix Astragali Membranacei (*Huang Qi*), Rhizoma Cimicifugae (*Sheng Ma*), mix-fried Radix Glycyrrhizae (*Zhi Gan Cao*), etc. Herbs which strengthen the spleen and transform dampness are: Fructus Amomi (*Sha Ren*), Radix Auklandiae (*Mu Xiang*), Fructus Amomi Cardamomi (*Bai Dou Kou*), Fructus Crataegi (*Shan Zha*), Massa Medica Fermentata (*Shen Qu*), Szechuan Cortex Magnoliae Officinalis (*Chuan Hou Po*), Herba Agastachis Seu Pogostemi (*Huo Xiang*), Herba Eupatorii Fortunei (*Pei Lan*), etc.

2. *Bu Shen*
Supplementing the Kidneys

The kidneys are the prenatal root and are the center of regulation of all the organs in the body. Insufficiency of kidney essence may lead to the deficiency and emptiness of all the other organs. Concomitantly, deficiency and emptiness of any of the other viscera may lead to deficiency detriment of the kidneys. In clinical practice, AIDS usually presents insufficiency of either kidney yin or kidney yang or emptiness of both kidney yin *and* yang. Modern research has shown that, in kidney deficient patients, metabolism, cellular immunity, and humoral immunity are all lower than in normal persons. Also, experiments have proven that TCM's kidney-supplementing method can improve human immunity and maintain disease resistance within the body.

Kidney emptiness is usually divided into emptiness of kidney yin and emptiness of kidney yang. It has been reported that herbs supplementing kidney yin can improve the body's immunity and prolong the survival of antibodies. While herbs warming and supplementing kidney yang can excite the nerves and humoral reaction, strengthen body resistance, and promote the formation of antibodies. In clinical practice, the commonly used herbs for supplementing kidney yin include: Prepared Radix Rehmanniae (*Shu Di*), processed Radix Polygoni Multiflori (*Zhi Shou Wu*), Fructus Ligustri Lucidi (*Nu Zhen*

Zi), Fructus Lycii Chinensis (*Gou Qi Zi*), Plastrum Testudinis (*Gui Ban*), Carapax Amydae Sinensis (*Bie Jia*), Fructus Schizandrae Chinensis (*Wu Wei Zi*), Tuber Asparagi Cochinensis (*Tian Men Dong*), Rhizoma Anemarrhenae (*Zhi Mu*), Herba Ecliptae Prostratae (*Han Lian Cao*), and Ramulus Loranthi Seu Visci (*Sang Ji Sheng*). Herbs which warm the kidneys and assist yang are: Herba Epimedii (*Yin Yang Huo*), Radix Morindae Officinalis (*Ba Ji Tian*), Rhizoma Curculiginis Orchioidis (*Xian Mao*), Herba Cistanchis (*Rou Cong Rong*), Cordyceps Sinensis (*Dong Chong Xia Cao*), Fructus Psoraleae Corylifoliae (*Bu Gu Zhi*), Herba Cynomorii Songarici (*Suo Yang*), Cortex Cinnamomi (*Rou Gui*), Semen Cnidii Monnieri (*She Chuang Zi*), Radix Dipsaci (*Xu Duan*), Cortex Eucommiae Ulmoidis (*Du Zhong*), etc.

Because yin and yang are interdependent, herbs which warm and supplement kidney yang are usually used with herbs which nourish and supplement kidney yin. This is because when yang grows, yin is strong and when yin grows, yang is strong. As stated in *Jing Yue Quan Shu (The Complete Writings of [Zhang] Jing-yue)*:

> In order to supplement yang, find yang within yin. Yin must help yang in order for it to grow without limit. In order to supplement yin, find yin within yang. Yang must promote yin for its spring to be inexhaustible.

B. *Qing Re Jie Du*
Clearing Heat & Resolving Toxins

AIDS is an infectious disease brought on by invasion of pestilential toxic evils. In the initial stage, there are usually some signs of heat or pathological changes due to emptiness and hot toxins existing simultaneously. In the advanced stage, pestilential toxic evils hide internally. Accumulation may transform into heat or viscera and bowels vacuity and decline may be accompanied by invasion of external evils. This usually results in the accumulation and stagnation of hot toxins. Hot toxins accumulating internally then present or manifest on the surface. In such cases, treatment should focus on clearing heat and resolving toxins so as to support the righteous and eliminate evil. When evils are expelled and the righteous is calm, the goal may be obtained. Experiments have proven that herbs which clear heat and resolve toxins are also anti-inflammatory, antiviral, and antibacterial.

Though some clinically effective heat-clearing herbs have no demonstrable antiviral or antibacterial effect, they may work by improving body immunity. However, AIDS is basically a righteous emptiness and heat-clearing, toxin-resolving herbs are usually bitter and cold. Bitter, cold (herbs) are contraindicated in *xu lao* or empty taxation diseases. Therefore, herbs which are bitter and cold should be combined with those that are sweet and warm so that support of the righteous is combined with elimination of evil. This prevents dispelling evils therapy from damaging the righteous. Recovery can only be obtained by a combination of supporting the righteous and eliminating evil so as to eliminate evil without harming the righteous.

The commonly used herbs in clinical practice for clearing heat and resolving toxins include: Flos Lonicerae Japonicae (*Jin Yin Hua*), Fructus Forsythiae Suspensae (*Lian Qiao*), Folium Daqingye (*Da Qing Ye*), Radix Isatidis Seu Baphicacanthi (*Ban Lan Geng*), Herba Cum Radice Taraxici Mongolici (*Pu Gong Ying*), Herba Cum Radice Violae Yedoensis (*Zi Hua Di Ding*), Spica Prunellae Vulgaris (*Xia Gu Cao*), Herba Cum Radice Houttuyniae Cordatae (*Yu Xing Cao*), Radix Scutellariae Baicalensis (*Huang Qin*), Rhizoma Coptidis Chinensis (*Huang Lian*), Cortex Phellodendri (*Huang Bai*), Radix Sophorae Flavescentis (*Ku Shen*), Calculus Bovis (*Niu Huang*), and Fructus Bruceae Javanicae (*Ya Dan Zi*).

Herbs with tumor-inhibiting functions are: Rhizoma Paridis Polyphyllae (*Quan Shen*), Herba Galli Aparinis (*Zhu Yang Yang*), Herba Pteridis Multifidae (*Feng Wei Cao*), Herba Scutellariae Barbatae (*Ban Zhi Lian*), Herba Oldenlandiae Diffusae (*Bai Hua She She Cao*), Herba Duchesneae Indicae (*She Mei*), and Radix Lithospermi Seu Arnebiae (*Zi Cao*). Because AIDS patients usually have complications due to yeast and fungal infection, some antimycotic herbs, such as Radix Sophorae Flavescentis (*Ku Shen*), Cortex Dictamni (*Bai Xian Pi*), Radix Et

Rhizoma Rhei (*Da Huang*), Rhizoma Belamcandae (*She Gan*), Radix Pulsatillae Chinensis (*Bai Tou Weng*), Radix Platycodi Grandiflori (*Jie Geng*), Herba Cum Radice Houttuyniae Cordatae (*Yu Xing Cao*), Flos Caryophylli (*Ding Xiang*), Pericarpium Punicae Granati (*Shi Liu Pi*), Cortex Phellodendri (*Huang Bai*), and Radix Scutellariae Baicalensis (*Huang Qin*), may also be used.

C. *Huo Xue Hua Yu*
Quickening the Blood & Transforming Stasis

The *Nei Jing* says, "Qi and blood not harmonious, thus 100 diseases change and arise." Qi and blood are the basic materials of the body's life. The transportation and movement of blood and fluids depends on the pushing movement of the qi. In other words,

If qi moves, blood moves. If qi stagnates, blood becomes static.

Because qi and blood are deficient and empty in those with AIDS, it may not be strong enough to push and move the circulation of blood and fluids. Therefore, there is usually qi stagnation and blood stasis in AIDS causing concretions and conglomerations, accumulations and gatherings and all kinds of malignant tumors. Thus the treatment of the above should quicken the blood and transform stasis.

It has now been proven that herbs quickening the blood and transforming stasis can reduce capillary permeability, are anti-inflammatory, activate the absorption of inflammation, and regulate the immune system. In clinical practice, the commonly used herbs for quickening the blood and transforming stasis include: Radix Angelicae Sinensis (*Dang Gui*), Radix Ligustici Wallichii (*Chuan Xiong*), Radix Rubrus Paeoniae Lactiflorae (*Chi Shao*), Semen Pruni Persicae (*Tao Ren*), Flos Carthami Tinctorii (*Hong Hua*), Radix Salviae Miltiorrhizae (*Dan Shen*), Tuber Curcumae (*Yu Jin*), Radix Pseudoginseng (*San Qi*), Rhizoma Corydalis Yanhusuo (*Yan Hu Suo*), Resina Olibani (*Ru Xiang*), Resina Myrrhae (*Mo Yao*), Rhizoma Sparganii (*San Leng*), Rhizoma Curcumae Zedoariae (*E Zhu*), Squama Manitis Pentadactylis

(*Chuan Shan Jia*), Hirudo (*Shui Zhi*), Feces Trogopterori Seu Pteromi (*Wu Ling Zhi*), Semen Vaccariae Segetalis (*Wang Bu Liu Xing*), and Spina Gleditchiae Sinensis (*Zao Ci*). Due to hypoimmunity, AIDS is usually accompanied by various sorts of tumors. Some tumor-combatting herbs for quickening the blood and cracking stasis which can be used are: Rhizoma Sparganii (*San Leng*), Rhizoma Curcumae Zedoariae (*E Zhu*), Bulbus Shancigu (*Shan Ci Gu*), Cantharides (*Ban Mao*), Semen Strychnotis Nux-vomicae (*Ma Qian Zi*), Rhizoma Corydalis Yanhusuo (*Yan Hu Suo*), Radix Semiaquilegiae (*Tian Kui Zi*), Hirudo (*Shui Zhi*), Tabanus (*Meng Chong*), and Herba Solani Nigri (*Long Kui*).

In the course of treating AIDS, attention should be paid that herbs for quickening the blood and transforming stasis are not used unnecessarily. They should only be used judiciously on the basis of such signs as a dark complexion, rough skin, fixed pain, an ecchymotic tongue, and a grating/astringent pulse. Due to the weakness of AIDS patients, some herbs for supplementing the qi, such as Radix Codonopsis Pilosulae (*Dang Shen*), Radix Astragali Membranacei (*Huang Qi*), and Rhizoma Atractylodis Macrocephalae (*Bai Zhu*), should accompany herbs for eliminating blood stasis in order to quicken the blood by activating the flow of qi. In short, only the combination of draining and supplementing will result in the desired effect. If drainage is overused, the case may become serious.

D. *Ruan Jian San Jie*
Softening the Hard & Scattering Nodulation

Phlegm is both a pathological product caused by viscera and bowel deficiency and vacuity and a further cause of disease. AIDS patients often have spleen emptiness with water dampness stopped up inside. Or, epidemic toxic evil heat may first stew the fluids and humors and change them into kernels of phlegm. Phlegm follows the ascent and descent of qi and may congeal under the skin resulting in the arisal of phlegm nodulation (*tan he*), scrofula, and lymphadenopathy. This should be treated by transforming phlegm, softening the hard, and scattering

43

nodulation. The accumulation and stagnation of phlegm turbidity may block the flow of qi. Therefore, when phlegm-transforming and softening the hard herbal medicinals are used, typically herbs for regulating the flow of qi are added, such as Pericarpium Citri Reticulatae (*Chen Pi*), Folium Citri (*Ju Ye*), Fructus Aurantii (*Zhi Ke*), Pericarpium Arecae (*Da Fu Pi*), Rhizoma Cyperi Rotundi (*Xiang Fu*), Fructus Citri Sacrodactylis (*Fo Shou Gan*), Pericarpium Citri Reticulatae Viride (*Qing Pi*), Rhizoma Corydalis Yanhusuo (*Yan Hu Suo*), Radix Auklandiae (*Mu Xiang*), and Flos Pruni Mume (*Lu E Mei*).

Research has proven that herbs which transform phlegm and soften the hard not only are able to soften the hard and scatter nodulation, disperse and eliminate swelling and lumps but also drain fire and purge heat, inhibit viruses, and break down tumors. Also, because evil turbid phlegm usually follows the ascent and descent of qi and is very changeable, it is important in treatment to separate clear from turbid, evil from righteous, emptiness from fullness, and whether to transform phlegm and soften the hard before, after, or at the same time as supporting and assisting the righteous all in order to effectively support the righteous and eliminate evil. The commonly used herbs in clinical practice for transforming phlegm, softening the hard, and scattering nodulation include: Spica Prunellae Vulgaris (*Xia Gu Cao*), Herba Sargassii (*Hai Zao*), Pumice (*Hai Fu Shi*), Gecko Swinhoa (*Bi Hu*), Bulbus Shancigu (*Shan Ci Gu*), Bulbus Fritillariae (*Bei Mu*), Thallus Algae (*Kun Bu*), Fructus Forsythiae Suspensae (*Lian Qiao*), Bombyx Batryticatus (*Bai Jiang Can*), Rhizoma Arisaematis (*Nan Xing*), Rhizoma Pinelliae Ternatae (*Ban Xia*), and Radix Semiaquilegiae (*Tian Kui Zi*).

4

Ai Zi Bing Ge Qi De Bian Zheng Zhi Liao

The *Bian Zheng* Treatment of the Various Stages of AIDS

The basic methodology of TCM is the treatment of disease based on the discrimination of patterns. This should be applied according to the principle of viewing the body as a whole. This means "searching for the cause of the disease from its manifestations" and "treating the disease having searched for its root." In clinical practice, one must consider the cause of the disease, its disease mechanism, and its course and development as well as its signs and symptoms. One must examine the patient using TCM's four diagnoses combined with tongue and pulse signs. These then should all be differentiated according to the theory of the eight principles and the viscera and bowels. Finally, one analyzes and summarizes the results in order to decide upon the correct treatment principles and methods and, thus, the choice of prescriptions and medicinals.

Based on AIDS' clinical manifestations, an analysis of its pathology, and modern medicine's division of the various stages of AIDS, patients in these various stages should be treated according to the following discrimination of patterns.

I. *Ai Zi Bing Qian Fu Qi*
AIDS Latent Stage, *i.e.*, Asymptomatic Virus-carrying Stage

In the initial stage of AIDS infection, there is usually a transient period of weight loss, fatigue, night sweats, diarrhea, lymphadenopathy, and other infectious symptoms. Then the patient recovers and enters the asymptomatic, virus-carrying stage. In this stage, the virus usually has a latency period of up to 5 years without any signs of disease. However, such virus carriers can infect other people through blood transfusion and other ways and hence are dangerous. This stage can only be diagnosed by blood tests of human immune deficiency virus antibodies if positive or if T_4 lymphocytes are reduced and the T_4/T_8 ratio is reversed.

According to traditional Chinese medical theory, infection by the AIDS virus is usually the result of deficiency and vacuity of righteous qi and invasion by viral evils. Therefore, its main treatment principles are to support the righteous and eliminate evil. In this latent stage, pathological changes are mostly due to the struggle between the deficient and vacuous righteous qi and the pestilential evils hidden internally. However, these are difficult to discover because they are asymptomatic. Nonetheless, this stage can be diagnosed based on a modern medical analysis of physical changes (such as in the blood) as well as changes in the tongue and pulse. Thus treatment can be administered based on a combination of pattern discrimination and disease discrimination.

A. *Qi Xue Kui Xu Xing*
Qi & Blood Deficiency & Vacuity Pattern

Clinical manifestations: Typically, the patient is markedly physically weak and their ability to resist disease is low. Or, because of lowered immunity and bodily vacuity and weakness, there is commonly epidemic taxation, impaired memory, insomnia, etc.

Treatment principles: Support the righteous and secure the root, regulate and supplement qi and blood

Guiding formula: *Ren Shen Gui Pi Wan Jia Jian*

Medicinals: Radix Panacis Ginseng (*Ren Shen*), Radix Angelicae Sinensis (*Dang Gui*), Radix Astragali Membranacei (*Huang Qi*), Rhizoma Atractylodis Macrocephalae (*Bai Zhu*), Sclerotium Poriae Cocos (*Fu Ling*), Semen Zizyphi Spinosae (*Suan Zao Ren*), Radix Polygalae Tenuifoliae (*Yuan Zhi*), Radix Auklandiae (*Mu Xiang*), Arillus Euphoriae Longanae (*Long Yan Rou*), uncooked Rhizoma Zingiberis (*Sheng Jiang*), Fructus Zizyphi Jujubae (*Da Zao*), and mix-fried Radix Glycyrrhizae (*Zhi Gan Cao*)

Formula Explanation: In this formula, the ingredients of *Si Jun Zi Tang* supplement and fortify the spleen. When the spleen and stomach promote transportation, qi and blood automatically arise. Radix Astragali Membranacei and Radix Angelicae Sinensis are added to form *Dang Gui Bu Xue Tang* in order to boost qi to engender the blood. Arillus Euphoriae Longanae, Semen Zizyphi Spinosae, and Radix Polygalae Tenuifoliae enrich heart blood and quiets the spirit. Radix Auklandiae rectifies the qi and arouses the spleen. Uncooked Rhizoma Zingiberis and Fructus Zizyphi Jujubae regulate and harmonize the contructive and defensive. Thus the goal of securing the root is achieved.

When taken over a prolonged period of time, this formula supplements the righteous and improves human immunity. In this formula, Radix Panacis Ginseng activates the hypophyseal-adrenocortical system, improves immunity, prevents allergic reactions, and stimulates hemopoiesis. It also improves the transformation of lymphoblasts. Radix Astragali Membranacei also improves human immunity. And, according to studies in Japan, mix-fried Radix Glycyrrhizae with its chief ingredient, glycyrrhizin, inhibits the growth of the AIDS virus and cytomorphosis.

Additions & Subtractions (*Jia Jian*): For those with vacuity of kidney yin, add Fructus Ligustri Lucidi(*Nu Zhen Zi*), Fructus Lycii Chinensis (*Gou Qi Zi*), and Herba Ecliptae Prostratae (*Han Lian Cao*). For those with kidney yang vacuity, add Herba Epimedii (*Yin Yang Huo*), Radix Mori Albindae Officinalis (*Ba Ji Tian*), Cortex Eucommiae Ulmoidis (*Du Zhong*), and Herba Cistanchis (*Rou Cong Rong*). For those with vacuous lung qi, add Gelatinum Corii Asini (*E Jiao*) and Bulbus Lilii (*Bai He*). And for those with lung yin vacuity, add Tuber Ophiopogonis Japonicae (*Mai Dong*), uncooked Radix Rehmanniae (*Sheng Di*), and Radix Glehniae Littoralis (*Sha Shen*).

Selected acupuncture/moxibustion points: *Zu San Li* (St 36)тх, *Shen Shu* (Bl 23)т, *Da Zhui* (GV 14)т, & *Guan Yuan* (CV 4)ᴀ

Formula rationale: *Zu San Li* is the sea point of the foot *yang ming* channel. Because the *yang ming* has a lot of qi and a lot of blood, needling using supplementing method and moxibustion can balance and regulate the spleen and stomach and supplement and boost the postnatal root. *Guan Yuan* is the meeting point of the *ren mai* and the three leg yin channels and governs the yin of the entire body. Moxaing this point supplements and boosts the prenatal root, boosts the qi, and secures the root. *Shen Shu* (Bl 23) is the back *shu* point of the kidney channel. Supplementing it fills kidney essence. *Da Zhui* (GV 14) is a channel point on the *du mai* and the meeting point of all 6 yang channels. It is able to supplement the yang qi of the entire body. It also upbears yang and boosts the qi. Thus its use assists in supporting the righteous and eliminating evil.

Additions & Subtractions: If the body is more inclined to kidney vacuity, add moxibustion at *Ming Men* (GV 4) to help warm and supplement the life gate fire or and supplement the kidneys and bank the source. For predominance of spleen vacuity, add supplementing *Pi Shu* (Bl 20) and moxa *Zhong Wan* (CV 12) to help supplement the spleen, boost the qi, and fortify the stomach and center. For predominance of lung vacuity, add supplementing *Fei Shu* (Bl 13) and moxa *Gao Huang* (Bl 43) to help supplement the lungs and boost the qi, warm the lungs and secure vacuity.

Note: This book uses the following symbols regarding acupuncture/moxibustion techniques.

Even supplementation, even drainage method: |
Needling with supplementation method: ⊤
Needling with drainage method: ⊥
Bleeding: ↓
Moxa with cones: ▲
Moxa with roll: x
Needling with supplementation plus cone moxa: ⊤▲
Needling with supplementation plus roll moxa: ⊤x

B. *Gan Yu Xing*
Liver Depression Pattern

Clinical manifestations: Patients are usually introverted. As soon as being diagnosed, there is typically and immediately depression and other emotional changes, such as fright and loneliness, chest oppression, sighing, lateral costal distention and fullness, etc.

Treatment principles: Supplement the righteous and secure the root, course the liver and resolve toxins

Guiding formula: *Fu Zheng Jie Yu Wan*

Medicinals: Radix Panacis Ginseng (*Ren Shen*), Radix Astragali

Membranacei (*Huang Qi*), Radix Bupleuri (*Chai Hu*), Rhizoma Pinelliae Ternatae (*Ban Xia*), Rhizoma Cyperi Rotundi (*Xiang Fu*), Fructus Aurantii (*Zhi Ke*), Radix Scutellariae Baicalensis (*Huang Qin*), uncooked Rhizoma Zingiberis (*Sheng Jiang*), Fructus Zizyphi Jujubae (*Da Zao*), & mix-fried Radix Glycyrrhizae (*Zhi Gan Cao*)

Formula Explanation: In this formula, Radix Panacis Ginseng and Radix Astragali Membranacei supplement the middle and boost the qi, support the righteous and bank the root. Radix Bupleuri, Rhizoma Cyperi Rotundi, and Fructus Aurantii course the liver, move the qi, and resolve depression, therefore rousing the essence spirit or mind. Rhizoma Pinelliae Ternatae harmonizes the stomach and downbears turbidity. It also aids Radix Scutellariae Baicalensis in clearing heat and resolving toxins. Uncooked Rhizoma Zingiberis, Fructus Zizyphi Jujubae, and mix-fried Radix Glycyrrhizae regulate the constructive and defensive and harmonize the preceding medicinals. They also support and assist the righteous qi. According to Japanese studies, *Xiao Chai Hu Tang*, which is included in this formula, has several immune-regulating functions and especially induces an increase of T_4 lymphocytes and thus improves cellular immunity.

Selected acupuncture/moxibustion points: *Zu San Li* (St 36) тx, *Guan Yuan* (CV 4)ᴀ, *Shen Shu* (Bl 23)т, *Tai Chong* (Liv 3)⊥, & *Shen Men* (Ht 7)⊥

Formula rationale: Needling and afterwards moxaing *Zu San Li* supplements and boosts the postnatal root and hence strengthens disease resistance. Moxaing *Guan Yuan* supplements and boosts prenatal essence. *Shen Shu* supplements and boosts kidney yin and kidney yang, thus filling kidney essence and automatically balancing yin and yang. Adding drainage of *Tai Chong* is able to course the liver and rectify the qi, move the qi and resolve depression. Draining *Shen Men* tranquilizes the heart and quiets the spirit. If heart spirit is calm, the above symptoms are automatically eliminated.

C. *Zheng Xie Xiang Chi Xing*
Righteous & Evil Locked in Stalemate Pattern

Clinical manifestations: Physically, the patient is comparatively strong and unyielding. After infection, there are usually no symptoms. The tongue and pulse are also like a normal person's.

Treatment principles: Support the righteous and secure the root, dispel evils and resolve toxins

Guiding formula: *Fu Zheng Jie Du Wan Jia Jian*

Medicinals: Radix Codonopsis Pilosulae (*Dang Shen*), Radix Astragali Membranacei (*Huang Qi*), Rhizoma Atractylodis Macrocephalae (*Bai Zhu*), Sclerotium Poriae Cocos (*Fu Ling*), Radix Sophorae Flavescentis (*Ku Shen*), Rhizoma Smilacis Glabrae (*Tu Fu Ling*), Folium Daqingye (*Da Qing Ye*), Herba Oldenlandiae Diffusae (*Bai Hua She She Cao*), Fructus Forsythiae Suspensae (*Lian Qiao*), Rhizoma Coptidis Chinensis (*Huang Lian*), mix-fried Radix Glycyrrhizae (*Zhi Gan Cao*)

Formula explanation: In this formula, *Si Jun Zi Tang* fortifies the spleen and boosts the qi, supplements the qi and enriches the blood. Radix Astragali Membranacei supplements the center and boosts the qi. Rhizoma Smilacis Glabrae and Folium Daqingye resolve toxins. Radix Sophorae Flavescentis and Rhizoma Coptidis Chinensis clear and discharge internal accumulation of epidemic evils. And Fructus Forsythiae Suspensae and Herba Oldenlandiae Diffusae clear heat and resolve toxins. The above medicinals when used together are able to support the righteous and dispel evils.

It is reported that every year about 30% of HIV positive patients progress to ARC. The above decoction can improve the immunity of patients and inhibit multiplication of the virus, thus controlling or slowing down this change for the worse.

Selected acupuncture/moxibustion points: *Zu San Li* (St 36)ᴀ, *Guan Yuan* (CV 4)ᴀ, *Da Zhui* (GV 14)⊤, *Qu Chi* (LI 11)|, & *He Gu* (LI 4)|

Formula rationale: Moxaing *Zu San Li* supplements and boosts qi and blood as well as banks and supplements the postnatal. Moxaing *Guan Yuan* warms and supplements the lower source. Use of supplementing technique at *Da Zhui* rouses yang qi, boosts the qi, and secures the exterior. These three points used together supplement and aid the righteous qi, bank the root, and secure the source. Even supplementation/even drainage of *Qu Chi* and *He Gu* frees the flow of the channels and quickens the network vessels, resolves toxins and scatters evils. Therefore, they are able to dispel evils and resolve toxins.

Note: In clinical practice, *Zu San Li, Guan Yuan, Da Zhui,* and other such points are able to stimulate the righteous qi of the human body and hence strengthen disease resistance. As the *Qian Jin Fang (Prescriptions [Worth] a 1,000 [Pieces of] Gold)* says:

> Ordinarily, when officials travel to Wu and Shu, they moxa their body constantly at both of the body's *San (Li)* and keep these blistered for the length of their errand. Thus fatigue and taxation, warm (diseases) and malaria, and toxic qi are not able to afflict them.

Therefore, patients in this stage should keep on taking Chinese medicinals and getting acupuncture/moxibustion treatment to improve the immunity of the body and so inhibit the increase in viruses and thus control their pathology.

II. *Ai Zi Bing Xiang Guan Zong He Zheng Qi* AIDS-related Complex (ARC)

In patients who progress from asymptomatic, latent viral infection to AIDS-related complex or ARC, there may be fever, sweating, aversion to cold, emaciation, poor appetite, prolonged diarrhea, lymphadenopathy, and other similar symptoms. This is usually followed by serious symptoms of righteous qi debility and vacuity and the appearance of vacuity detriment of the viscera and bowels. Usually, at the beginning, only one viscus is deficient and vacuous. Gradually this involves other viscera. The pathology continues to develop day by day and this hastens the occurrence of complications. In this stage, the pathological symptoms are those of debility and emptiness of the viscera and bowels and qi and blood and the expression of internal, hidden, epidemic toxic evils on the outside. At this stage, the main symptoms are a feeling of fever on the outside and aversion to cold. The treatment principles are to eliminate evil and support the righteous. Because the clinical symptoms are mainly those of vacuity detriment, the main treatment principles are to supplement and boost.

A. Vacuity of The Righteous Plus External Invasion

In the initial stage of AIDS, one commonly sees fever accompanied by other superficial or vacuous symptoms. Treatment should primarily eliminate evil and support the righteous. Because of differences in various types of evil qi, both the specific disease manifestations and specific treatments (for these manifestations) likewise should vary.

1. *Yin Xu Wai Gan Fa Re Xing*
Yin Vacuity with External Invasion & Fever Pattern

Clinical manifestations: Typically there is lack of strength in the whole body, heat in the hands, feet, and heart, low back and knee soreness and weakness, seminal emission, premature ejaculation, palpitations, and insomnia. Then appear low fever, fear of wind, *i.e.*, drafts, thirst, sore throat, cough with little phlegm, chest pain, lymphadenopathy in the back of the neck, underarms, and groin, etc., a red tongue with scant fur, and a floating, fine, and rapid pulse.

Treatment principles: Nourish yin and transform phlegm, clear heat and resolve the exterior

Guiding formula: *Wei Ru Tang* plus *Yang Yin Qing Fei Tang Jia Jian*

Medicinals: Rhizoma Polygonati Odorati (*Yu Zhu*), Radix Cynanchi (*Bai Wei*), Radix Platycodi Grandiflori (*Jie Geng*), Herba Menthae Haplocalycis (*Bo He*), Semen Praeparatus Sojae (*Dan Dou Chi*), uncooked Radix Rehmanniae (*Sheng Di*), Tuber Ophiopogonis Japonicae (*Mai Dong*), Bulbus Fritillariae Cirrhosae (*Chuan Bei Mu*), Radix Scrophulariae Ningpoensis (*Yuan Shen*), Radix Isatidis Seu Baphicacanthi (*Ban Lan Geng*), Folium Daqingye (*Da Qing Ye*), Flos Lonicerae Japonicae (*Yin Hua*), Concretio Silicae Bambusae (*Tian Zhu Huang*), Radix Glycyrrhizae (*Gan Cao*)

Formula explanation: In this formula, Herba Menthae Haplocalycis, Semen Praeparatus Sojae, and Radix Platycodi Grandiflori course the exterior, discharge heat, and lightly diffuse lung qi. Rhizoma Polygonati Odorati and Tuber Ophiopogonis Japonicae nourish yin and engender fluids, thus assisting the origin of sweat. Radix Cynanchi and Radix Rehmanniae clear heat and enrich yin. Radix Scrophulariae Ningpoensis enriches yin, moistens dryness, clears the lungs, and resolves toxins. Flos Lonicerae Japonicae, Folium Daqingye, and Radix Istadis Seu Baphicacanthi clear heat and resolve toxins, thus expelling pestilential evils. And Bulbus Fritillariae Cirrhosae and Concretio Silcea Bambusae clear heat and transform phlegm, disperse scrofula and scatter nodulation.

Selected acupuncture/moxibustion points: *Lie Que* (Lu 7)⊥, *Zhi Zheng* (SI 7)⊥, *Fei Shu* (Bl 13)⊤, *Feng Chi* (GB 20)⊥, *Fu Liu* (Ki 7)⊤, & *San Yin Jiao* (Sp 6)⊤

Formula rationale: Draining the network point of the lung channel, *Lie Que*, eliminates wind and resolves the exterior, diffuses the lungs and transforms phlegm. When drained, the network point of the hand *tai yang* channel, *Zhi Zheng*, plus *Feng Chi* eliminate wind, scatter cold, and resolve external evils from the *tai yang*. Supplementing *Fei Shu* is able to supplement and boost lung qi. Supplementing *Fu Liu* is capable of nourishing yin and enriching fluids. *San Yin Jiao* is the meeting point of the foot three yin. It is used to nourish yin and enrich the blood.

2. *Qi Xu Wai Gan Fa Re Xing*
Qi Vacuity with External Invasion & Fever Pattern

Clinical manifestations: Extreme lack of strength, spontaneous perspiration, voice tiny and faint, lassitude of the spirit, weary and unable to work, whole body uncomfortable, palpitations and shortness of breath on exertion, fever aggravated by taxation, or slight aversion to wind (*i.e.,* draft) and cold, cough with scant phlegm, body pain, or lymphadenopathy, a pale tongue with thin fur, and a floating, forceless pulse

Treatment principles: Boost the qi and secure the exterior, transform phlegm and resolve toxins

Guiding formula: *Yu Ping Feng San Jia Wei*

Medicinals: Radix Astragali Membranacei (*Huang Qi*), Rhizoma Atractylodis Macrocephalae (*Bai Zhu*), Radix Panacis Ginseng (*Ren Shen*), Radix Ledebouriellae Sesloidis (*Fang Feng*), Sclerotium Poriae Cocos (*Fu Ling*), Flos Lonicerae Japonicae (*Yin Hua*), Fructus Forsythiae Suspensae (*Lian Qiao*), Radix Platycodi Grandiflori (*Jie Geng*), Bulbus Fritillariae Cirrhosae (*Chuan Bei Mu*), Radix Isatidis Seu Baphicacanthi (*Ban Lan Geng*), Radix Glycyrrhizae (*Gan Cao*)

Formula explanation: Radix Astragali Membranacei boosts the qi and secures the exterior. It is combined with Rhizoma Atractylodis Macrocephalae which fortifies the spleen and boosts the qi. (The ingredients of) *Si Jun Zi Tang* supplement the center and boost the qi, endender the qi and blood, and thus secure the root. Flos Lonicerae Japonicae, Fructus Forsythiae Suspensae, and Radix Isatidis Seu

55

Baphicacanthi clear heat and resolve toxins. Radix Platycodi Grandiflori and Bulbus Fritillariae Cirrhosae resolve toxins, transform phlegm, and scatter nodulation. Radix Ledebouriellae Sesloidis eliminates wind evils and relieves the exterior. And Radix Glycyrrhizae regulates and harmonizes the preceding medicinals.

If there is external invasion of wind cold with extreme aversion to cold, one may use *Shen Su Yin Jia Jian* to boost the qi and secure the exterior.

Medicinals: Radix Panacis Ginseng (*Ren Shen*), Folium Perillae Frutescentis (*Su Ye*), Radix Puerariae (*Ge Geng*), Radix Peucedani (*Qian Hu*), Rhizoma Pinelliae Ternatae (*Ban Xia*), Fructus Aurantii (*Zhi Ke*), Sclerotium Poriae Cocos (*Fu Ling*), Pericarpium Citri Reticulatae (*Chen Pi*), Radix Platycodi Grandiflori (*Jie Geng*), Radix Auklandiae (*Mu Xiang*), Radix Glycyrrhizae (*Gan Cao*)

Formula explanation: Radix Panacis Ginseng and Sclerotium Poriae Cocos fortify the spleen and boost the qi, thus eliminating evil. Folium Perillae Frutescentis, Radix Puerariae, and Radix Peucedani eliminate wind, relieve the exterior, and scatter cold. Rhizoma Pinelliae Ternatae, Fructus Aurantii, and Radix Platycodi Grandiflori diffuse the lungs and rectify the qi, transform phlegm and stop coughing, disperse scrofula and scatter nodulation. Pericarpium Citri Reticulatae and Radix Auklandiae rectify the qi and harmonize the middle. And Radix Glycyrrhizae regulates and harmonizes the preceding medicinals.

Selected acupuncture/moxibustion points: *Lie Que* (Lu 7)⊥, *Ying Xiang* (LI 20)⊤, *Zu San Li* (St 36) ▵, *Feng Chi* (GB 20)|, *He Gu* (LI 4)⊥, & *Fei Shu* (Bl 13)⊤

Formula rationale: *Lie Que* is the network point of the lung channel and is able to diffuse the lungs and relieve the exterior. In combination with *Ying Xiang*, it scatters external evils. Moxaing *Zu San Li* fortifies the spleen and nourishes the stomach, supplements the center and boosts the qi. Adding drainage of *Feng Chi* eliminates wind and scatters cold. Purging *He Gu* courses and disinhibits the *yang ming*, eliminates wind, and relieves the exterior. And *Fei Shu* is chosen to supplement and boost lung qi and to secure and guard the righteous qi.

3. *Qi Xu Yang Ming Re Cheng Xing*
Qi Vacuity, Heat Accumulating in the *Yang Ming* Pattern

Clinical manifestations: High fever not relieved by sweating, thirst, vexation and agitation, disquietude, *i.e.,* restlessness, cough, chest pain, constipation, emaciation, body habitually vacuous, weary, unable to work, lack of strength, both eyes red, a red tongue, and a rapid, forceless pulse

Treatment principles: Boost the qi and engender fluids, clear heat and resolve toxins

Guiding formula: *Bai Hu Jia Ren Shen Tang Jia Jian*

Medicinals: Gypsum Fibrosum (*Shi Gao*), Radix Panacis Ginseng (*Ren Shen*), Rhizoma Anemarrhenae (*Zhi Mu*), Flos Lonicerae Japonicae (*Yin Hua*), Pulvis Indigonis (*Qing Dai*), Sclerotium Poriae Cocos (*Fu Ling*), Bulbus Fritillariae Cirrhosae (*Chuan Bei Mu*), Pericarpium Citri Reticulatae (*Chen Pi*), Cortex Radicis Mori Albi (*Sang Bai Pi*), Radix Scutellaraie Baicalensis (*Huang Jin*), Radix Glycyrrhizae (*Gan Cao*)

Formula explanation: Gypsum Fibrosum is acrid, sweet, and very cold and clears lung and stomach heat. It is combined with Rhizoma Anemarrhenae which enrichen yin, clears heat, and eliminates vexation. Radix Panacis Ginseng boosts the qi and secures the root. Flos Lonicerae Japonicae, Fructus Forsythiae Suspensae, and Pulvis Indigonis clear heat and resolve toxins. Sclerotium Poriae Cocos fortifies the spleen and eliminates dampness. Cortex Radicis Mori Albi, Bulbus Fritillariae Cirrhosae, Pericarpium Citri Reticulatae, and

Radix Scutellariae Baicalensis clear heat, transform phlegm, and stop coughing. And Radix Glycyrrhizae regulates and harmonizes the preceding medicinals.

If there is high fever with delirium aggravated at night, this is due to heat evils internally trapped in the pericardium. (For this,) one can use *An Gong Niu Huang Wan* to clear heat and open the portals. If the heat is not relieved and there are skin rashes and eruptions or severe delirium at night, a dark red tongue and a fine, rapid pulse, this is heat entering the constructive and blood aspects.

Treatment principles: Clear heat and resolve toxins, cool the blood and scatter stasis

Guiding formula: *Qing Ying Tang Jia Wei*

Medicinals: Cornu Rhinocerotis[1] (*Xi Jiao*), uncooked Radix Rehmanniae (*Sheng Di*), Cortex Radicis Moutan (*Dan Pi*), Rhizoma Coptidis Chinensis (*Huang Lian*), Herba Lophatheri Gracilis (*Dan Zhu Ye*), Tuber Ophiopogonis Japonicae (*Mai Dong*), Flos Lonicerae Japonicae (*Yin Hua*), Fructus Forsythiae Suspensae (*Lian Qiao*), Radix Scrophulariae Ningpoensis (*Yuan Shen*), Radix Rubrus Paeoniae Lactiflorae (*Chi Shao*)

Formula explanation: Cornu Rhinocerotis cools the blood, clears heat, and resolves toxins from the constructive aspect. Uncooked Radix Rehmanniae enriches yin, clears heat, and cools the blood. Radix Rubrus Paeoniae Lactiflorae and Cortex Radicis Moutan clear heat and cool the blood, quicken the blood and scatter stasis. Tuber Ophiopogonis Japonicae, Herba Lophatheri Gracilis, and Radix

---

[1]

Blue Poppy Press does not endorse the use of any endangered species for medicinal purposes. Other ingredients may be substituted for Cornu Rhinocerotis in this formula or in any other where it is mentioned.

Scrophulariae Ningpoensis clear heat, resolve toxins, and eliminate pestilential toxic evils.

Selected acupuncture/moxibustion points: *Chi Ze* (Lu 5)⊥, *Yu Ji* (Lu 10)↓, *Qu Chi* (LI 11)⊥, *Nei Ting* (St 44)⊥, *Zu San Li* (St 36)⊤, & *Da Zhui* (GV 14)⊥

Formula rationale: The spring point of the hand *tai yin* channel, *Yu Ji*, combined with the sea point, *Chi Ze*, clears and discharges heat evils. The sea point of the *yang ming, Qu Chi*, clears and resolves the *yang ming*. Adding the spring point of the foot *yang ming, Nei Ting*, clears heat and engenders fluids. The *du mai* is the sea of all yang vessels. Therefore, *Da Zhui* is chosen to secure and guard the righteous and course and clear heat evils. *Zu San Li* boosts the qi, fortifies the spleen, and clears heat.

If there is delirium due to high fever, drain *Ren Zhong* (GV 26) and bleed the *Shi Xuan* to open the portals, arouse the spirit, and discharge evil heat. For heat which has entered the constructive and blood with skin rashes and eruptions, drain *Xue Hai* (Sp 10) and bleed the twelve well points to clear the constructive and cool the blood.

B. Chronic Vacuity Patterns

Based on clinical experience, during the intermediate or intermediate-advanced stage or after appropriate treatment, the manifestations of the initial stage, such as fever and aversion to cold, diminish. These are then replaced by chronic vacuity symptoms. These include vacuity of qi, blood, yin or yang, and of the five viscera. Typically, vacuity of one viscus affects all the others during the course of development of this disease. This leads to a gradual worsening of the case and complications. During this stage, treatment should mainly entail supplementing methods. The main patterns in this stage are vacuity of the kidneys and spleen. The spleen is the postnatal root of qi and blood production. The kidneys are the prenatal root and residence of source yin and yang. Therefore, supplementation of the kidneys and spleen are the main treatment methods at this stage.

1. *Fei Qi Xu Xing*
Lung Qi Vacuity Pattern

Clinical manifestations: Disinclination to speak, fear of wind or draft, spontaneous perspiration, cough, shortness of breath, sometimes fever, sometimes chills, liability to catch cold, facial color pale, a pale tongue, and a weak or deep, fine, forceless pulse.

Treatment principles: Supplement and boost the lung qi

Guiding formula: *Bu Fei Tang Jia Jian*

Medicinals: Radix Panacis Ginseng (*Ren Shen*), Radix Astragali Membranacei (*Huang Qi*), Prepared Radix Rehmanniae (*Shu Di*), Fructus Schizandrae Chinensis (*Wu Wei Zi*), Radix Asteris Tatarici (*Zi Wan*), Sclerotium Poriae Cocos (*Fu Ling*), Rhizoma Atractylodis Macrocephalae (*Bai Zhu*), Cortex Radicis Mori Albi (*Sang Bai Pi*), mix-fried Radix Glycyrrhizae (*Zhi Gan Cao*)

Formula explanation: Radix Panacis Ginseng and Radix Astragali Membranacei supplement the lungs, boost the qi, and secure the exterior. (The ingredients of) *Si Jun Zi Tang* boost the qi and fortify the spleen, thus banking earth to engender metal. Radix Asteris Tatarici and Cortex Radicis Mori Albi transform phlegm, downbear qi, and stop coughing. Prepared Radix Rehmanniae and Fructus Schizandrae Chinensis boost the kidneys, secure the source, and astringe the lungs. Taken as a whole, this formula has the ability to supplement and boost lung qi, secure the exterior, and stop coughing.

Selected acupuncture/moxibustion points: *Fei Shu* (Bl 13)⊤, *Gao Huang* (Bl 43)⌂, *Bai Hui* (GV 20) ⊤, *Zu San Li* (St 36)⊤, & *Qi Hai* (CV 6)⌂

Formula rationale: *Fei Shu* is chosen to supplement and boost lung qi. Because *Gao Huang* is the main point for treating vacuity taxation, it is moxaed to warm the lungs and supplement and boost. *Bai Hui* boosts the qi and ascends yang. *Zu San Li* supplements the center and boosts the qi, thus cultivating earth to generate metal. Moxaing *Qi Hai* is used to boost the qi, secure the exterior, and supplement and boost kidney qi.

2. *Fei Qi Yin Liang Xu Xing*
Lung Qi & Yin Dual Vacuity Pattern

Clinical manifestations: Lassitude of the spirit, lack of strength, face white, shortness of breath, disinclination to speak, cough with little phlegm or phlegm mixed with blood, tidal fever and night sweats or spontaneous perspiration, dry mouth and throat, lack of sleep, a red tongue with scant fur, and a fine, rapid, forceless pulse

Treatment principles: Boost the qi and nourish yin, clear dryness and moisten the lungs

Guiding formula: *Sheng Mai San* plus *Qing Zao Jiu Fei Tang Jia Jian*

Medicinals: Tuber Ophiopogonis Japonicae (*Mai Dong*), Folium Mori Albi Albi (*Sang Ye*), Gypsum Fibrosum (*Shi Gao*), Gelatinum Corii Asini (*E Jiao*), Radix Glycyrrhizae (*Gan Cao*), Radix Panacis Ginseng (*Ren Shen*), Fructus Schizandrae Chinensis (*Wu Wei Zi*), Folium Eriobotryae Japonicae (*Pi Pa Ye*), Semen Pruni Armeniacae (*Xing Ren*)

Formula explanation: Radix Panacis Ginseng supplements the lungs, boosts the qi, and engenders fluids. It is combined with Tuber Ophiopogonis Japonicae, which nourishes yin and clears heat. Fructus Schizandrae Chinensis astringes the lungs and stops sweating. These three medicinals together boost the qi and support the righteous, nourish yin and engender fluids. Folium Mori Albi Albi lightly diffuses lung qi. Gypsum Fibrosum clears lung dry heat. Gelatinum Corii Asini

61

moistens the lungs and enriches yin. And Semen Pruni Armeniacae and Folium Eriobotryae Japonicae clear and discharge lung heat.

Selected acupuncture/moxibustion points: *Fei Shu* (Bl 13)⊤, *Fu Liu* (Ki 7)|, *Gao Huang* (Bl 43)▵, *Chi Ze* (Lu 5)⊥, *Tai Xi* (Ki 3)⊤, & *Da Zhui* (GV 14)|

Formula rationale: *Fei Shu* is chosen to supplement and boost lung qi. Even supplementation and drainage of *Fu Liu* enriches yin and engenders fluids. Moxaing *Gao Huang* is a main point for supplementing vacuity taxation. *Chi Ze* is drained to clear the lung channel of vacuous heat, stop cough, and level asthma. *Tai Xi* used with supplementing method nourishes and supplements lung and kidney yin. *Da Zhui* with even supplementation and drainage is chosen because it is able to aid yang, clear heat, and expel evils.

3. *Pi Qi Xu Xing*
Spleen Qi Vacuity Pattern

Clinical manifestations: A sallow yellow facial complexion, scanty appetite, lassitude of the spirit, lack of strength, loose stools, spontaneous perspiration, a pale tongue with thin fur, and a vacuous pulse

Treatment principles: Supplement the middle, boost the qi, and fortify the spleen

Guiding formula: *Jia Wei Si Jun Zi Tang*

Medicinals: Radix Panacis Ginseng (*Ren Shen*), Radix Astragali Membranacei (*Huang Qi*), Rhizoma Atractylodis Macrocephalae (*Bai Zhu*), mix-fried Radix Glycyrrhizae (*Zhi Gan Cao*), Sclerotium Poriae Cocos (*Fu Ling*), Semen Dolichoris Lablab (*Bian Dou*)

Formula explanation: Radix Panacis Ginseng supplements the center and boosts the qi. Rhizoma Atractylodis Macrocephalae, sweet and bitter, fortifies the spleen and dries dampness. Radix Astragali Membranacei combined with Radix Panacis Ginseng greatly supplements the source qi, thus securing the root. Adding Sclerotium Poriae Cocos with its sweet, bland (flavor) seeps dampness, thus strengthening the spleen. Semen Dolichoris Lablab, sweet and warm, fortifies the spleen and transforms dampness. Mix-fried Radix Glycyrrhizae, sweet, relaxes and harmonizes the center. Used together, the above medicinals supplement the center, boost the qi, and fortify the spleen. Therefore, they are able to disperse this pathocondition.

Selected acupuncture/moxibustion points: *Zu San Li* (St 36)⊤, *Pi Shu* (Bl 20)⊤, *Zhong Wan* (CV 12)▵, & *Tian Shu* (St 25)|

Formula rationale: Supplementing *Zu San Li* is chosen to fortify the spleen and boost the qi, warm the center and harmonize the stomach. *Pi Shu* is able to supplement the spleen and boost the stomach. Moxaing *Zhong Wan* strengthens the stomach and supplements the center, regulates and regulates the stomach and intestines. *Tian Shu* is on the foot *yang ming* stomach channel. It is also the front *mu* point of the large intestine. Even supplementation and drainage of it can stop diarrhea. Thus defecation is automatically regulated.

4. *Pi Xu Shi Zu Xing*
Spleen Vacuity, Damp Obstruction Pattern

Clinical manifestations: Lassitude of the spirit, lack of strength, emaciation, no desire for food and drink, even nausea, vomiting, abdominal distention and fullness, a sallow yellow facial complexion, diarrhea, a pale tongue with a white, slimy fur, and an vacuous, relaxed pulse

Treatment principles: Fortify the spleen and boost the qi, harmonize the stomach and transform fluids

Guiding formula: *Shen Ling Bai Zhu San Jia Jian*

63

Medicinals: Radix Panacis Ginseng (*Ren Shen*), Rhizoma Atractylodis Macrocephalae (*Bai Zhu*), Sclerotium Poriae Cocos (*Fu Ling*), Radix Dioscoreae Oppositae (*Shan Yao*), mix-fried Radix Glycyrrhizae (*Zhi Gan Cao*), Semen Dolichoris Lablab (*Bian Dou*), Semen Nelumbinis Nuciferae (*Lian Zi Rou*), Semen Coicis Lachryma-jobi (*Yi Ren*), Mix-fried Radix Glycyrrhizae Amomi (*Sha Ren*), Rhizoma Pinelliae Ternatae (*Ban Xia*), Pericarpium Citri Reticulatae (*Chen Pi*)

Formula explanation: Radix Codonopsis Pilosulae (*Dang Shen*) warms and supplements the center and boosts the qi. Rhizoma Atractylodis Macrocephalae, which is sweet and bitter, fortifies the spleen and dries dampness. Sclerotium Poriae Cocos, due to its sweet, bland flavor, seeps dampness and fortifies the spleen. Radix Dioscoreae Oppositae and Semen Nelumbinis Nuciferae boost the qi and fortify the spleen, harmonize the stomach and stop thirst. Adding Semen Dolichoris and Semen Coicis Lachryma-jobi seeps dampness and fortifies the spleen. Mix-fried Radix Glycyrrhizae, sweet, boosts the qi and harmonizes the center. Mix-fried Radix Glycyrrhizae Amomi harmonizes the stomach and assists the spleen, rectifies the qi and loosens the chest. Adding Rhizoma Pinelliae Ternatae and Pericarpium Citri Reticulatae rectifies the qi and harmonizes the stomach as well as downbears counterflow and stops vomiting.

Selected acupuncture/moxibustion points: *Zhong Wan* (CV 12)△, *Tian Shu* (St 25)|, *Pi Shu* (Bl 20)⊤, *Zu San Li* (St 36)⊤, *Yin Ling Quan* (Sp 9)⊥

Formula rationale: Moxaing *Zhong Wan* is able to warm the stomach, harmonize the center, and eliminate dampness. *Pi Shu* is chosen to supplement the spleen and boost the stomach. *Tian Shu* with even supplementation and drainage is chosen for its ability to regulate the stomach and intestines, stop diarrhea and disperse distention. Supplementing *Zu San Li* is used to fortify the spleen, boost the qi, and supplement the center. Draining *Yin Ling Quan* disinhibits water and moves dampness. When dampness is eliminated, spleen/stomach transportation is promoted.

5. *Pi Xu Xue Kui Xing*
Spleen Vacuity, Blood Deficient Pattern

Clinical manifestations: A pale white facial complexion, dizziness, blurred vision, lassitude of the spirit, lack of strength, heart palpitations, shortness of breath, no desire for food and drink, a pale tongue with white fur, and a fine, weak pulse

Treatment principles: Fortify the spleen, boost the qi, and nourish the blood

Guiding formula: *Ba Zhen Tang*

Medicinals: Radix Panacis Ginseng (*Ren Shen*), Rhizoma Atractylodis Macrocephalae (*Bai Zhu*), Sclerotium Poriae Cocos (*Fu Ling*), Radix Angelicae Sinensis (*Dang Gui*), Radix Ligustici Wallichii (*Chuan Xiong*), Radix Albus Paeoniae Lactiflorae (*Bai Shao*), Prepared Radix Rehmanniae (*Shu Di*), mix-fried Radix Glycyrrhizae (*Zhi Gan Cao*), uncooked Rhizoma Zingiberis (*Sheng Jiang*), Fructus Zizyphi Jujubae (*Da Zao*)

Formula explanation: In this formula, *Si Jun Zi Tang* supplements the qi and fortifies the spleen. When the spleen and stomach promote transportation, food and drink are automatically regulated. Radix Angelicae Sinensis and Radix Albus Paeoniae Lactiflorae nourish the blood and harmonize the constructive. Radix Ligustici Wallichii activates the blood and moves the qi. Mix-fried Radix Glycyrrhizae boosts the qi and harmonizes the middle. Uncooked Rhizoma Zingiberis and Fructus Zizyphi Jujubae regulate and harmonize the spleen and stomach. Taken as a whole, this formula boosts the qi and fortifies the spleen. When qi and blood are both supplemented, this pathocondition is automatically regulated.

Selected acupuncture/moxibustion points: *Zu San Li* (St 36)т, *Pi Shu* (Bl 20)т, *San Yin Jiao* (Sp 6)т, *Ge Shu* (Bl 17)т, & *Xue Hai* (Sp 10)т

65

Formula rationale: Using *Zu San Li* with supplementating technique supplements and boosts the qi and blood, boosts the qi and fortifies the spleen, thus banking and supplementing of the postnatal root. *Pi Shu* is chosen to fortify the spleen and boost the stomach, thus qi and blood are automatically generated. *San Yin Jiao* supplements and boosts yin essence, fortifies the spleen and nourishes the blood. Supplementing *Xue Hai* is chosen to nourish and generate the blood, fortify the spleen and conserve the blood. *Ge Shu* is the *hui* reunion point of the blood. Supplementing it nourishes and engenders the blood.

6. *Pi Xu Xia Xiang Xing*
Vacuous Spleen Falls Downward Pattern

Clinical manifestations: Prolonged diarrhea which will not recover, lassitude of the spirit, lack of strength, shortness of breath, faint, feeble voice, dizziness, blurred vision or spontaneous perspiration, emaciation, diminished food intake, a distended and sagging sensation in the lower abdomen or signs of prolapse of the internal viscera, a pale tongue with white fur, and an vacuous, soft, forceless pulse.

Treatment principles: Supplement the center and fortify the spleen, upbear yang and lift the fallen

Guiding formula: *Bu Zhong Yi Qi Tang Jia Jian*

Medicinals: Radix Panacis Ginseng (*Ren Shen*), Radix Astragali Membranacei (*Huang Qi*), Radix Angelicae Sinensis (*Dang Gui*), Rhizoma Atractylodis Mcrocephalae (*Bai Zhu*), Rhizoma Cimicifugae (*Sheng Ma*), Radix Bupleuri (*Chai Hu*), Pericarpium Citri Reticulatae (*Chen Pi*), mix-fried Radix Glycyrrhizae (*Zhi Gan Cao*)

Formula explanation: Radix Astragali Membranacei supplements the center and boosts the qi, upbears yang, secures the exterior, and stops sweating. Radix Codonopsis Pilosulae (*Dang Shen*), Rhizoma Atractylodis Macrocephalae, and mix-fried Radix Glycyrrhizae are added to boost the qi and fortify the spleen. This automatically fortifies the spleen/stomach's formation of righteous qi. Pericarpium Citri Reticulatae rectifies the qi and transforms stasis. Radix Angelicae Sinensis supplements the blood and harmonizes the constructive. Using a little Rhizoma Cimicifugae and Radix Bupleuri strengthens the function of Radix Panacis Ginseng and Radix Astragali Membranacei in upbearing yang and lifting the fallen. Hence the downward falling is thus lifted and raised.

Selected acupuncture/moxibustion points: *Zu San Li* (St 36)⊤, *Guan Yuan* (CV 4)⊤, *Bai Hui* (GV 20)⊤, & *Pi Shu* (Bl 20)⊤

Formula rationale: The head is the reunion of yang. Therefore, *Bai Hui* is chosen to ascend the yang and boost the qi and thus the sunken is lifted. *Guan Yuan* is chosen to supplement the qi and secure the fallen. Supplementing *Zu San Li* results in boosting the qi and strengthening the spleen, balancing the stomach, intestines, and qi mechanism *vis à vis* transportation and transformation. This automatically results in stopping diarrhea. *Pi Shu* is added because of its ability to additionally fortify the spleen and boost the qi.

7. *Gan Yu Pi Xu Xing*
Liver Depression, Spleen Vacuity Pattern

Clinical manifestations: A lusterless complexion, diminished desire for food, abdominal distention, loose stools or borborygmus, diarrhea, emotional depression, frequent sighing, restlessness, lateral costal distention and oppression, lack of sleep, heart vexation, a pale tongue with white fur, and a wiry, fine pulse

Treatment principles: Course the liver and resolve depression, rectify the qi and fortify the spleen

Guiding formula: *Xiao Yao San Jia Jian*

Medicinals: Radix Bupleuri (*Chai Hu*), Rhizoma Cyperi Rotundi (*Xiang Fu*), Fructus Aurantii (*Zhi Ke*), Pericarpium Citri Reticulatae (*Chen Pi*), Radix Angelicae Sinensis (*Dang Gui*), Sclerotium Poriae Cocos (*Fu Ling*), Rhizoma Atractylodis Macrocephalae (*Bai Zhu*), Radix Albus Paeoniae Lactiflorae (*Bai Shao*), mix-fried Radix Glycyrrhizae (*Zhi Gan Cao*)

Formula explanation: Radix Bupleuri courses the liver and resolves depression. Rhizoma Cyperi Rotundi and Fructus Aurantii when added to Radix Bupleuri strengthen the function of rectifying the qi and coursing the liver. Pericarpium Citri Reticulatae moves the qi, fortifies the spleen, and transforms dampness. Radix Angelicae Sinensis and Radix Albus Paeoniae Lactiflorae nourish the blood and supplement the liver. Rhizoma Atractylodis Macrocephalae boosts the qi and fortifies the spleen. Sclerotium Poriae Cocos seeps dampness and fortifies the spleen. And mix-fried Radix Glycyrrhizae regulates and harmonizes the preceding medicinals. The combination of the above formula courses the liver and resolves depression, nourishes the blood, boosts the qi, and fortifies the spleen.

Selected acupuncture/moxibustion points: *Zu San Li* (St 36)⊤, *Qi Hai* (CV 6)⊥, *Shan Zhong* (CV 17)⊥, *Tai Chong* (Liv 3)⊥, *Shen Men* (Ht 7)⊥, & *San Yin Jiao* (Sp 6)⊤

Formula rationale: *Zu San Li* is chosen to supplement and boost qi and blood, regulate and regulate the spleen and stomach. Draining *Shan Zhong* loosens the chest and rectifies the qi, moves the qi and courses the liver. Draining *Tai Chong* courses the liver, levels the *chong*, and downbears counterflow. Draining *Shen Men* settles the heart and quiets the spirit. Supplementing *San Yin Jiao* fortifies the spleen and supplements and boosts yin essence. And draining *Qi Hai* moves the qi and scatters stasis, courses and resolves liver depression.

8. *Xin Pi Liang Xu Xing*
Heart/Spleen Dual Vacuity Pattern

Clinical manifestations: Heart palpitations, lack of sleep, profuse dreaming, anxiety, vexation, agitation, disquietude, *i.e.*, restlessness, entire body lack of strength, dizziness, hands and feet chilly, diarrhea or loose stools, appetite diminished, itching skin, facial rashes or face ashen and white, a pale tongue with white, greasy fur, and a deep, forceless pulse

Treatment principles: Boost the qi and supplement the blood, fortify the spleen and nourish the heart

Guiding formula: *Gui Pi Tang Jia Jian*

Medicinals: Radix Astragali Membranacei (*Huang Qi*), Rhizoma Atractylodis Macrocephalae (*Bai Zhu*), Radix Codonopsis Pilosulae (*Dang Shen*), Radix Angelicae Sinensis (*Dang Gui*), Radix Polygalae Tenuifoliae (*Yuan Zhi*), Sclerotium Pararadicis Poriae Cocos (*Fu Shen*), Semen Zizyphi Spinosae (*Suan Zao Ren*), Prepared Radix Rehmanniae (*Shu Di*), Radix Auklandiae (*Mu Xiang*), Pericarpium Citri Reticulatae (*Chen Pi*), Os Draconis (*Sheng Long Gu*), mix-fried Radix Glycyrrhizae (*Zhi Gan Cao*), Arillus Euphoriae Longanae (*Long Yan Rou*)

Formula explanation: In this formula, *Si Jun Zi Tang* fortifies the spleen. Radix Astragali Membranacei and Radix Angelicae Sinensis form *Dang Gui Bu Xue Tang* which supplements the qi and engenders blood. Radix Auklandiae and Pericarpium Citri Reticulatae fortify the spleen and rectify the qi in order to prevent supplementation causing stasis. Radix Polygalae Tenuifoliae, Arillus Euphoriae Longanae, and Sclerotium Pararadicis Poriae Cocos nourish the heart and calm the spirit. Os Draconis suppresses yang and hence quiets the spirit. The above medicinals together are able to supplement and boost qi and blood, fortify the spleen and nourish the heart, as well as calm the spirit.

69

Selected acupuncture/moxibustion points: *Zu San Li* (St 36)⊤, *Xin Shu* (Bl 15)⊤, *Pi Shu* (Bl 20)⊤, *Shen Men* (Ht 7)⊥, *Nei Guan* (Per 6)⊥, & *Ge Shu* (Bl 17)⊥

Formula rationale: Supplementing *Xin Shu* supplements heart qi, settles the heart spirit, and nourishes heart blood. *Zu San Li* supplements and boosts the spleen and stomach and engenders qi and blood. *Pi Shu* supplements the spleen and boosts the stomach. *Shen Men* is the source point of the heart channel. When drained, it quiets the spirit. Draining the network point of the pericardium channel, *Nei Guan*, frees and disinhibits the heart network vessels, quiets the spirit, and tranquilizes fright. Supplementing *Ge Shu* transforms and engenders yin and blood.

9. *Pi Shen Qi Xu Xing*
Spleen/kidney Qi Vacuity Pattern

Clinical manifestations: Bodily emaciation, fatigue, inability to work, lack of strength, spontaneous perspiration, epigastric and abdominal lumps and fullness, diarrhea, borborygmus, low back and knee soreness and weakness, possible whole body edema, dizziness, tinnitus, seminal emission, impotence, a somber white facial complexion, a weak, faint, feeble voice, a pale tongue with white fur, and a weak pulse

Treatment principles: Boost the qi and fortify the spleen, supplement the kidneys and assist yang

Guiding formula: *Bu Zhong Yi Qi Tang* plus *Jin Gui Shen Qi Wan*

Medicinals: Radix Astragali Membranacei (*Huang Qi*), Radix Codonopsis Pilosulae (*Dang Shen*), Rhizoma Atractylodis Macrocephalae (*Bai Zhu*), Pericarpium Citri Reticulatae (*Chen Pi*), Rhizoma Cimicifugae (*Sheng Ma*), Radix Bupleuri (*Chai Hu*), Prepared Radix Rehmanniae (*Shu Di*), Fructus Corni Officinalis (*Shan Zhu Yu*), Radix Dioscoreae Oppositae (*Shan Yao*), Cortex

Radicis Moutan (*Dan Pi*), Sclerotium Poriae Cocos (*Fu Ling*), Rhizoma Alismatis (*Ze Xie*), Radix Lateralis Praeparatus Aconiti Carmichaeli (*Fu Zi*), Cortex Cinnamomi (*Rou Gui*), Semen Cuscutae (*Tu Si Zi*)

Formula explanation: Radix Astragali Membranacei boosts the qi and secures the root. *Si Jun Zi Tang* boosts the qi and fortifies the spleen. Pericarpium Citri Reticulatae rectifies the qi. The addition of a little Rhizoma Cimicifugae and Radix Bupleuri boosts the qi and ascends the yang. Prepared Radix Rehmanniae and Fructus Corni Officinalis enrich and supplement kidney essence. Radix Dioscoreae Oppositae, sweet and warm, fortifies the spleen. Adding a little Cortex Radicis Moutan and Rhizoma Alismatis regulates the liver, spleen, and kidneys, and a little Radix Lateralis Praeparatus Aconiti Carmichaeli and Cortex Cinnamomi warms kidney yang to absorb kidney qi. Used together, these medicinals boost the qi and fortify the spleen, supplement the kidneys and assist yang.

Selected acupuncture/moxibustion points: *Shen Shu* (Bl 23)⊤, *Qi Hai* (CV 6)▵, *Zu San Li* (St 36)⊤, & *Bai Hui* (GV 20)x

Formula rationale: Moxaing *Qi Hai* is able to greatly supplement the source qi and rectifies the qi mechanism in the lower burner, thus filling kidney qi. Supplementing *Shen Shu* boosts the kidneys and secures the root. Because the *yang ming* channel has a lot of qi and a lot of blood, *Zu San Li* supplements and boosts qi and blood. Moxaing *Bai Hui* upbears yang and boosts the qi, supplements and boosts kidney qi.

10. *Shen Jing Bu Zu Xing*
Kidney Essence Insufficiency Pattern

Clinical manifestations: Falling, fading hair, loose teeth, tinnitus, deafness, essence sppirit dull or absent-minded, forgetful, lassitude of the spirit, movement slow or sluggish or mind dull and stupid, lower extremities feeble, weak, and without strength, vision unclear, slow, dull, inappropriate responses, a pale tongue, and a weak pulse.

Treatment principles: Fill and supplement kidney essence, boost qi and nourish blood

Guiding formula: *He Che Zai Zao Wan Jia Jian*

Medicinals: Herba Cistanchis (*Rou Cong Rong*), Tuber Asparagi Cochinensis (*Tian Dong*), uncooked Radix Rehmanniae (*Sheng Di*), Prepared Radix Rehmanniae (*Shu Di*), Cortex Eucommiae Ulmoidis (*Du Zhong*), Radix Mori Albindae Officinalis (*Ba Ji*), Gelatinum Corii Asini (*E Jiao*), Plastrum Testudinis (*Gui Ban*), Carapax Amydae Sinensis (*Bie Jia*), Radix Albus Paeoniae Lactiflorae (*Bai Shao*), Radix Glycyrrhizae (*Gan Cao*), Placenta Hominis (*Zi He Che*)

Formula explanation: Prepared Radix Rehmanniae enriches and supplements kidney essence. Placenta Hominis supplements and boosts essence and blood. Cortex Eucommiae Ulmoidis supplements the kidneys and strengthens the sinews and bones. Radix Mori Albindae Officinalis and Herba Cistanchis warm and supplement kidney yang. Radix Achyranthis Bidentatae enriches yin and strengthens the sinews and bones. Plastrum Testudinis and Carapax Amydae Sinensis supplement and boost kidney essence. Tuber Asparagi Cochinensis and Radix Rehmanniae enrich yin and engender fluids. And Radix Albus Paeoniae Lactiflorae and Radix Glycyrrhizae aid by harmonizing the middle.

Selected acupuncture/moxibustion points: *Shen Shu* (Bl 23)⊤, *Zu San Li* (St 36)⊤, *Guan Yuan* (CV 4)▵, *Tai Xi* (Ki 3)⊤, *San Yin Jiao* (Sp 6)⊤

Formula rationale: *Shen Shu* used with supplementating technique supplements the kidneys and boosts the essence. It is used to strengthen the lower and upper backs. *Zu San Li* supplements and boosts the spleen and stomach, thus engendering and transforming qi and blood. *Guan Yuan* is used with moxa method to warm and supplement the lower source, to supplement and boost the prenatal root, and to bank up and supplement kidney essence. *Tai Xi* enriches and supplements the yin and essence of the kidneys. And *San Yin Jiao*, being the meeting point of the foot three yin, boosts the essence and engenders blood when supplemented.

11. *Shen Yang Xu Xing*
Kidney Yang Vacuity Pattern

Clinical manifestations: Aversion to cold, cold limbs, facial color pale and white, clear, copious urine, seminal emission, impotence, diarrhea with undigested food or 5 AM diarrhea, a pale tongue with white fur, and a deep, slow pulse

Treatment principles: Warm and supplement kidney yang, simultaneously supplement essence and blood

Guiding formula: *You Gui Wan Jia Jian*

Medicinals: Prepared Radix Rehmanniae (*Shu Di*), Fructus Corni Officinalis (*Shan Zhu Yu*), Radix Dioscoreae Oppositae (*Shan Yao*), Fructus Lycii Chinensis (*Gou Qi Zi*), Cortex Eucommiae Ulmoidis (*Du Zhong*), Semen Cuscutae (*Tu Si Zi*), Radix Lateralis Praeparatus Aconiti Carmichaeli (*Fu Zi*), Cortex Cinnamomi (*Rou Gui*), Gelatinum Cornu Cervi (*Lu Jiao Jiao*)

Formula explanation: Prepared Radix Rehmanniae, sweet and warm, enriches the kidneys and fills the essence. Radix Lateralis Praeparatus Aconiti Carmichaeli and Cortex Cinnamomi warm and supplement kidney yang and eliminate cold. Fructus Corni Officinalis and Fructus Lycii Chinensis enrich the kidneys and nourish the liver. Radix Dioscoreae Oppositae and Radix Glycyrrhizae boost the qi and fortify the spleen. Cortex Eucommiae Ulmoidis supplements the liver and kidneys. Semen Cuscutae and Gelatinum Cornu Cervi supplement and boost kidney qi as well as warm the kidneys and fill the essence.

Selected acupuncture/moxibustion points: *Guan Yuan* (CV 4)ᴀ, *Ming Men* (GV 4)x, *Zu San Li* (St 36)ᴛ, *Shen Shu* (Bl 23)ᴛ, & *Tian Shu* (St 25)ᴀ

Formula rationale: Moxaing *Guan Yuan* warms and supplements the lower burner and supplements and boosts kidney yang. Moxaing *Ming Men* supplements the kidneys and warms yang. Supplementing *Zu San Li* supplements and boosts the spleen and stomach which are the postnatal root. Supplementing *Shen Shu* aids kidney yang. *Tian Shu* is a foot *yang ming* stomach channel point and also the front *mu* point of the large intestine. Moxaing it regulates and regulates the stomach and intestines.

12. *Pi Shen Yang Xu Xing*
Spleen/Kidney Yang Vacuity Pattern

Clinical manifestations: Facial edema, a pale white facial complexion, falling hair, itching skin, hands and feet not warm, aversion to cold and chilled extremities, low back, knee, and lower abdominal chilly pain, low back sore, legs weak, or diarrhea with undigested food, dizziness and vertigo, a pale tongue with glossy fur, and a fine, weak pulse

Treatment principles: Warm and supplement the spleen and kidneys

Guiding formula: *Fu Zi Li Zhong Tang* plus *You Gui Wan Jia Jian*

Medicinals: Radix Lateralis Praeparatus Aconiti Carmichaeli (*Fu Zi*), Cortex Cinnamomi (*Rou Gui*), Prepared Radix Rehmanniae (*Shu Di*), Radix Panacis Ginseng (*Ren Shen*), Rhizoma Atractylodis Macrocephalae (*Bai Zhu*), Rhizoma Desiccata Zingiberis (*Gan Jiang*), Radix Dioscoreae Oppositae (*Shan Yao*), Fructus Lycii Chinensis (*Gou Qi*), Semen Cuscutae (*Tu Si Zi*), Gelatinum Cornu Cervi (*Lu Jiao Jiao*), Fructus Corni Officinalis (*Shan Zhu Yu*), mix-fried Radix Glycyrrhizae (*Zhi Gan Cao*)

Formula explanation: Radix Panacis Ginseng supplements the center and boosts the qi. Rhizoma Atractylodis Macrocephalae and Radix Dioscoreae Oppositae boost the qi and fortify the spleen. Dry Rhizoma Zingiberis warms the center and supports the yang. Prepared Radix Rehmanniae enriches and supplements kidney essence. Fructus Corni Officinalis and Fructus Lycii Chinensis enrich and supplement kidney yang. Semen Cuscutae and Gelatinum Cornu Cervi supplement and boost kidney essence. Mix-fried Radix Glycyrrhizae harmonizes the middle and regulates and harmonizes the preceding medicinals.

Selected acupuncture/moxibustion points: *Zu San Li* (St 36)⊤, *Guan Yuan* (CV 4)▵, *Pi Shu* (Bl 20)⊤, *Zhong Wan* (CV 12)▵, & *Shen Shu* (Bl 23)⊤x

Formula rationale: Supplementing *Zu San Li* fortifies the spleen and boosts the qi, supplements and boosts the postnatal. Moxaing *Guan Yuan* warms the kidneys and supplements and boosts the prenatal. *Pi Shu* is chosen to supplement and boost spleen yang. Moxaing *Zhong Wan* warms the middle and harmonizes the stomach, regulates and regulates the stomach and intestines, and thus stops diarrhea. *Shen Shu* is needled and then moxaed in order to warm and supplement kidney yang. Together, these points have the ability to warm and supplement the spleen and kidneys.

13. *Shen Yin Xu Xing*
Kidney Yin Vacuity Pattern

Clinical manifestations: Exhausted spirit, lack of strength, dizziness, tinnitus, lack of sleep, night sweats, and dry mouth and throat accompanied by low back and knee soreness and weakness, a red tongue with scant fur, and a deep, fine pulse

Treatment principles: Enrich and supplement kidney yin

Guiding formula: *Zuo Gui Wan Jia Jian*

Medicinals: Prepared Radix Rehmanniae (*Shu Di*), Fructus Lycii Chinensis (*Gou Qi*), Radix Dioscoreae Oppositae (*Shan Yao*), Fructus Corni Officinalis (*Shan Zhu Yu*), Gelatinum Cornu Cervi (*Lu Jiao Jiao*), Semen Cuscutae (*Tu Si Zi*), Radix Cyathulae (*Chuan Niu Xi*)

Formula explanation: Prepared Radix Rehmanniae enriches and supplements kidney yin. Fructus Corni Officinalis and Fructus Lycii Chinensis enrich yin and nourish the blood. Radix Dioscoreae Oppositae boosts the qi and fortifies the spleen. Radix Cyathulae enriches kidney yin and lures vacuous fire to return to its source. Semen Cuscutae and Gelatinum Cornu Cervi enrich and supplement kidney essence, thus supplementing the kidneys and filling the essence.

If yin vacuity is severe with bone steaming, tidal fever, night sweats, and nocturnal seminal emissions:

Treatment principles: Enrich yin and downbear fire

Guiding formula: *Zhi Bai Di Huang Wan*

Medicinals: Prepared Radix Rehmanniae (*Shu Di*), Fructus Corni Officinalis (*Shan Zhu Yu*), Radix Dioscoreae Oppositae (*Shan Yao*), Rhizoma Alismatis (*Ze Xie*), Cortex Radicis Moutan (*Dan Pi*), Sclerotium Poriae Cocos (*Fu Ling*), Rhizoma Anemarrhenae (*Zhi Mu*), Cortex Phellodendri (*Huang Bai*)

Formula explanation: In this formula, Prepared Radix Rehmanniae enriches and supplements kidney essence. Fructus Corni Officinalis enriches and nourishes the liver and kidneys. Radix Dioscoreae Oppositae supplements, boosts, and fortifies the spleen. Sclerotium Poriae Cocos blandly seeps dampness and fortifies the spleen. Rhizoma Alismatis clears and purges kidney fire and simultaneously prevents Prepared Radix Rehmanniae's enrichment (from being too) greasy. Cortex Radicis Moutan clears and discharges liver fire. And Rhizoma Anemarrhenae and Cortex Phellodendri clear lower burner damp heat, thus enriching yin and downbearing fire.

Selected acupuncture/moxibustion points: *Shen Shu* (Bl 23)⊤, *Tai Xi* (Ki 3)⊤, *San Yin Jiao* (Sp 6)⊤, *Zu San Li* (St 36)⊤, & *Shen Men* (Ht 7)⊥

Formula rationale: Supplementing *Shen Shu* is chosen to supplement the kidneys and boost essence in order to rebalance yin and yang. Supplementing *Tai Xi* enriches and supplements kidney yin and descends vacuous fire. *San Yin Jiao* is the meeting point of the foot three yin. Its supplementation is able to enrich yin and engender the blood. *Zu San Li* supplements and boosts the postnatal root and transforms and engenders qi and blood. *Shen Men* is the *yuan* source point of the heart channel. Draining it can tranquilize the heart and calm the spirit.

14. *Gan Shen Yin Xu Xing*
Liver/Kidney Yin Vacuity Pattern

Clinical manifestations: Dizziness, blurred vision, tinnitus, deafness, ideas not clear, facial color wan and sallow, lack of sleep, impaired memory, low fever in the afternoon or at night, dry mouth and throat, low back and knee soreness and weakness, slight pain in the lateral costal region, vexatious heat in the five hearts or centers, both cheeks flushed red, emaciation, night sweats, mental depression, vexation and agitation, a red tongue with scant fur, and a fine, rapid pulse

Treatment principles: Enrich and supplement the liver and kidneys, course the liver and rectify the qi

Guiding formula: *Yi Guan Jian* plus *Liu Wei Di Huang Wan*

Medicinals: Prepared Radix Rehmanniae (*Shu Di*), uncooked Radix Rehmanniae (*Sheng Di*), Radix Glehniae Littoralis (*Sha Shen*), Fructus Lycii Chinensis (*Gou Qi*), Tuber Ophiopogonis Japonicae (*Mai Dong*), Radix Angelicae Sinensis (*Dang Gui*), Cortex Radicis Moutan (*Dan Pi*), Fructus Corni Officinalis (*Shan Zhu Yu*), Radix Dioscoreae Oppositae (*Shan Yao*), Sclerotium Poriae Cocos (*Fu*

Ling), Fructus Zizyphi Jujubae (*Da Zao*), Fructus Meliae Toosendan (*Chuan Lian Zi*)

Formula explanation: Radix Rehmanniae enriches and supplements the liver and kidneys as well as clears heat. Prepared Radix Rehmanniae enriches the kidneys and fills the essence. Fructus Corni Officinalis and Fructus Lycii Chinensis enrich and nourish the liver and kidneys. Radix Glehniae Littoralis and Tuber Ophiopogonis Japonicae nourish yin and engender fluids. Radix Angelicae Sinensis enriches yin and nourishes the blood. Radix Dioscoreae Oppositae and Sclerotium Poriae Cocos boost the qi and fortify the spleen. Fructus Zizyphi Jujubae nourishes heart blood and quiets the spirit. Adding a little Fructus Meliae Toosendan courses and discharges liver qi.

Selected acupuncture/moxibustion points: *Shen Shu* (Bl 23)⊤, *Gan Shu* (Bl 18)⊤, *Tai Xi* (Ki 3)⊤, *Tai Chong* (Liv 3)⊥, & *Shen Men* (Ht 7)⊥

Formula rationale: *Shen Shu* is chosen to supplement and boost kidney essence. *Tai Xi* enriches and supplements kidney yin. Used together, they enrich the kidneys and boost yin, supplement the kidneys and generate water. Thus they control source yang. *Gan Shu* enriches liver yin. Draining *Tai Chong* makes liver yang lie low. *Shen Men* is the source point of the heart channel. Draining it tranquilizes the heart and quiets the spirit.

Note: Most patients die within 3 years of the onset of the ARC stage of this disease. Therefore, the control of this ARC stage is crucially important. The above decoctions are both antiviral and improve body immunity. They also control and reduce opportunistic infections and prevent the disease from worsening. Supporting the righteous decoctions and pills can be administered alternately with toxin-resolving medicinals and decoctions, thus both supporting the righteous and eliminating evil. Or, one may support the righteous first and then eliminate the evil. However, it should be pointed out that prolonged supplementation may cause fullness and retention in the spleen. Therefore, some spleen-arousing medicinals or digestion-motivating medicinals should be used, or one may administer *Xiang Sha Liu Jun Zi Wan* so as to achieve the goal of normal spleen/stomach function. Thus absorption is strengthened.

III. *Wan Quan Ai Zi Bing Qi*
Full Blown AIDS Stage

The pathological manifestations of patients in the full blown AIDS stage are extreme physical vacuity and weakness, extraordinary emaciation, and all sorts of opportunistic infections, such as *Pneumocystis carnii* pneumonia and toxoplasmosis, and various kinds of malignant tumors, such as Kaposi's sarcoma. During this stage, the immune system is usually greatly impaired and body resistance is extremely low. The viscera and bowels, qi and blood are extremely deficient and damaged. This bodily weakness and the tendency to opportunistic infections form a pernicious circle and may quickly worsen the case leading to death. In addition, during this stage of AIDS, stagnant qi, blood stasis, and phlegm turbidity evils mutually and abundantly bind and knot together. Righteous qi does not have the strength to combat evil. In turn, this can be the cause of these foregoing malignant transformations. Therefore, in treating patients in the full blown stage of AIDS, treatment should primarily be based on methods of rectifying the qi, quickening the blood, eliminating phlegm, and transforming turbidity. These should not be overlooked or neglected.

A. *Gan Zhi Xue Yu Xing*
Liver Stagnation, Blood Stasis Pattern

Clinical manifestations: A dark facial complexion, chest and lateral costal pain, masses in the hypochondrium or abdomen, extreme aching and pain, location of the pain immovable or fixed, emotional depression, dark purplish lips and nails, a dark purplish tongue or static spots, and a fine, choppy pulse

Treatment principles: Quicken the blood and transform stasis, rectify the qi and scatter nodulation

Guiding formula: *Ge Xia Zhu Yu Tang Jia Jian*

Medicinals: Semen Pruni Persicae (*Tao Ren*), Flos Carthami Tinctorii (*Hong Hua*), Radix Angelicae Sinensis (*Dang Gui*), Radix Ligustici Wallichii (*Chaun Xiong*), Feces Trogopterori Seu Pteromi (*Wu Ling Zhi*), Rhizoma Corydalis Yanhusuo (*Yan Hu Suo*), Rhizoma Cyperi Rotundi (*Xiang Fu*), Fructus Immaturus Aurantii (*Zhi Shi*), Radix Glycyrrhizae (*Gan Cao*)

Formula explanation: Radix Angelicae Sinensis nourishes and activates the blood. Radix Ligustici Wallichii, Semen Pruni Persicae, and Flos Carthami Tinctorii quicken the blood and transform stasis. Feces Trogopterori Seu Pteromi eliminates stasis and stops pain. Rhizoma Corydalis Yanhusuo eliminates stasis, rectifies the qi, and stops pain. Rhizoma Cyperi Rotundi and Fructus Immaturus Aurantii course the liver and resolve depression, loosen the chest and move the qi, since when the qi moves, the blood moves. Radix Glycyrrhizae regulates and harmonizes the preceding medicinals.

If blood stasis is severe and there are tumors and masses, add Rhizoma Sparganii (*San Leng*), Rhizoma Curcumae Zedoariae (*E Zhu*), Eupolyphagae Seu Ophistoplatiae (*Di Bie Chong*), etc. to break nodulation and move stasis, scatter nodulation and disperse masses.

Selected acupuncture/moxibustion points: *Shan Zhong* (CV 17)⊥, *Qi Hai* (CV 6)⊥, *He Gu* (LI 4)⊥, *Zhang Men* (Liv 13)⊥, *Xue Hai* (Sp 10)⊥, & *Ge Shu* (Bl 17)|

Formula rationale: Draining *Shan Zhong* loosens the chest and disinhibits the diaphragm, rectifies the qi and frees the network vessels. Draining *Qi Hai* moves the qi and scatters nodulation, rectifies the qi and moves the blood. Draining *He Gu* moves and activates the blood. Draining *Zhang Men* courses the liver and disinhibits the gallbladder, moves the qi and disperses accumulations. Draining *Xue Hai* activates the blood and transforms stasis. And even supplementation and drainage of *Ge Shu* nourishes and activates the blood.

B. *Tan Zhuo Zu Luo Xing*
Phlegm Turbidity Obstructing the Network Vessel Pattern

Clinical manifestations: Scrofulous lumps under the jaw, in the underarms, and inguinal regions, subcutaneous nodules of varying size, skin color normal, skin warmth not changed, a thick, slimy tongue fur, and a wiry, slippery pulse

Treatment principles: Soften the hard and scatter nodulation, resolve toxins and wash away phlegm

Guiding formula: *Xiao Luo Wan Jia Jian*

Medicinals: Radix Scrophulariae Ningpoensis (*Yuan Shen*), Concha Ostreae (*Mu Li*), Bulbus Fritillariae Thunbergii (*Zhe Mu*), Bulbus Shancigu (*Shan Ci Gu*), Rhizoma Pinelliae Ternatae (*Ban Xia*), Bombyx Batryticatus (*Jiang Can*), Spica Prunellae Vulgaris (*Xia Gu Cao*), Herba Sargassii (*Hai Zao*), Rhizoma Arisaematis (*Nan Xing*), Semen Sinapis Albae (*Bai Jie Zi*), Herba Oldenlandiae Diffusae (*Bai Hua She She Cao*), Tuber Dioscoreae Bulbiferae (*Huang Yao Zi*)

Formula explanation: In this formula, Bulbus Fritillariae Thunbergii, Concha Ostreae, and Herba Sargassii soften the hard and scatter nodulation. Bile-processed Rhizoma Arisaematis (*Dan Nan Xing*), Rhizoma Pinelliae Ternatae, and Semen Sinapis Albae disperse phlegm, scatter nodulation, disinhibit the blood, and free the network vessels. Tuber Dioscoreae Bulbiferae and Bulbus Shangcigu clear heat and resolve toxins as well as transform phlegm and scatter nodulation. Herba Sargassii transforms phlegm, scatters nodulation, and disinhibits water. Bombyx Batryticatus softens the hard and transforms phlegm, resolves toxins and scatters nodulation. And Herba Oldenlandiae Diffusae clears heat and resolves toxins.

Selected acupuncture/moxibustion points: *Feng Long* (St 40)⊥, *Shao Hai* (Ht 3)⊥, *Tian Jing* (TH 10)⊥, & *Yin Ling Quan* (Sp 9)⊥

Formula rationale: *Feng Long* is a *yang ming* channel point. Draining it fortifies the spleen and stomach and transforms phlegm. *Shao Hai* is the sea point of the hand *shao yin* heart channel. Draining it downbears heart fire and transforms phlegm turbidity. *Tian Jing* is an empirically proven point for the treatment of scrofula. And *Yin Ling Quan* fortifies the spleen and disinhibits dampness, thus dispersing the origin of phlegm engenderment.

C. *Shi Re Yong Sheng Xing*
Damp Heat Congested & Exuberant Pattern

Clinical manifestations: Fever, dry mouth, sore throat, eruption of mouth sores, possible diarrhea with loose, foul-smelling stools, lower limb ulcers, short, red urine, a red tongue with yellow, slimy fur, and a slippery, rapid pulse

Treatment principles: Clear heat and resolve toxins, disinhibit dampness and transform turbidity

Guiding formula: *Gan Lu Xiao Du Dan Jia Jian*

Medicinals: Talcum (*Hua Shi*), Herba Artemisiae Capillaris (*Yin Chen*), Radix Scutellariae Baicalensis (*Huang Qin*), Bulbus Fritillariae Thunbergii (*Zhe Bei*), Caulis Akebiae (*Mu Tong*), Herba Agastachis Seu Pogostemi (*Huo Xiang*), Fructus Forsythiae Suspensae (*Lian Qiao*), Rhizoma Belamcandae (*She Gan*), Radix Auklandiae (*Mu Xiang*), Fructus Amomi Cardamomi (*Bai Kou Ren*)

Formula explanation: Talcum clears heat and disinhibits dampness. Herba Artemisiae Capillaris and Caulis Akebiae clear heat and disinhibit dampness by expelling damp heat via urination. Radix Scutellariae Baicalensis clears heat and dries dampness. Fructus Forsythiae Suspensae clears heat and resolves toxins. Bulbus Fritillariae Thunbergii and Rhizoma Belamcandae disinhibit the throat and resolve toxins. Herba Menthae Haplocalycis (*Bo He*) and Herba Agasthachis Seu Pogostemi fragrantly transform turbidity, thus waking the spleen. Used together, these medicinals eliminate evil toxins and clear damp heat.

If hot toxins are prominent, add Flos Lonicerae Japonicae (*Yin Hua*), Herba Cum Radice Taraxaci Mongolici (*Pu Gong Ying*), and Folium Daqingye (*Da Qing Ye*) to clear heat and resolve toxins. If damp heat in the liver channel pouring down is prominent with blisters and itching of the external genitalia and ulceration of the lower limbs, use *Long Gan Xie Gan Tang Jia Jian* in order to clear liver/gallbladder fire and drain damp heat from the three burners. It is composed of: Radix Bupleuri (*Chai Hu*), Rhizoma Alismatis (*Ze Xie*), Semen Plantaginis (*Che Qian Zi*), Caulis Akebiae (*Mu Tong*), uncooked Radix Rehmanniae (*Sheng Di*), rootlets of Radix Angelicae Sinensis (*Dang Gui Wei*), Radix Scutellariae Baicalensis (*Huang Qin*), Radix Glycyrrhizae (*Gan Cao*).

Selected acupuncture/moxibustion points: *Da Zhui* (GV 14)⊥, *Yang Ling Quan* (GB 34)⊥, *Qu Chi* (LI 11)⊥, *Jie Xi* (St 41)⊥, *Wei Zhong* (Bl 40)↓, & *Da Ling* (Per 7)⊥

Formula rationale: Draining *Da Zhui* clears heat. *Yang Ling Quan* clears heat, resolves toxins, and disinhibits dampness. *Qu Chi* is chosen to clear heat and resolve toxins. Bleeding *Wei Zhong* eliminates evils and scatters stasis, thus expelling evil toxins. *Jie Xi* is chosen to clear and descend stomach fire and clear and purge yang heat. Draining *Da Ling* eliminates evil and scatters stasis, leads off qi and blood, and expels evil heat.

D. *Tan Re Yun Fei Xing*
Phlegm Heat Accumulating in the Lungs Pattern

Clinical manifestations: Cough with little or copious yellow, slimy phlegm, chest pain, a dry mouth with bitter taste, asthma, a yellow, slimy tongue fur, and a slippery, rapid pulse

Treatment principles: Clear heat and transform phlegm, stop cough and level asthma

Guiding formula: *Qing Qi Hua Tan Wan Jia Jian*

Medicinals: Fructus Trichosanthis Kirlowii (*Gua Lou Ren*), Rhizoma Pinelliae Ternatae (*Ban Xia*), Pericarpium Citri Reticulatae (*Chen Pi*), Radix Scutellariae Baicalensis (*Huang Qin*), Semen Pruni Armeniacae (*Xing Ren*), Fructus Aurantii (*Zhi Ke*), Sclerotium Poriae Cocos (*Fu Ling*), Rhizoma Praeparatus Cum Fellim Bovim Arisaematis (*Dan Nan Xing*), Cortex Radicis Mori Albi (*Sang Bai Pi*), Herba Cum Radice Houttuyniae Cordatae (*Yu Xing Cao*), etc.

Formula explanation: Rhizoma Praeparatus Cum Fellim Bovim Arisaematis clears heat and transforms phlegm. This is combined with Radix Scutellariae Baicalensis and Fructus Trichosanthis Kirlowii, which transform phlegm and clear heat. Pericarpium Citri Reticulatae and Fructus Aurantii rectify the qi and loosen the chest, thus eliminating phlegm. Sclerotium Poriae Cocos fortifies the spleen and seeps dampness. Semen Pruni Armeniacae diffuses the lungs, stops cough, and levels asthma. Rhizoma Pinelliae Ternatae dries dampness and transforms phlegm. Cortex Radicis Mori Albi drains the lungs and levels asthma. And Herba Cum Radice Houttuyniae Cordatae clears lung heat, transforms phlegm, and resolves toxins.

Selected acupuncture/moxibustion points: *Fei Shu* (Bl 13)⊥, *Chi Ze* (Lu 5)⊥, *Qu Chi* (LI 11)⊥, *Feng Long* (ST 40)⊥, & *Zhong Fu* (Lu 1)⊥

Formula rationale: *Chi Ze* is the lung channel water point. Combined with *Fei Shu*, it can drain the lungs and transform phlegm. *Qu Chi* clears heat and resolves toxins, thus downbearing phlegm fire. *Feng Long* is drained to transform phlegm and eliminate fire. And *Zhong Fu* is the front *mu* point of the lungs. Draining it clears the lungs and levels asthma.

E. *Tan Mi Xin Qiao Xing*
Phlegm Confounding the Heart Portals Pattern

Clinical manifestations: Dementia, slow responses, heart palpitations, dizziness, fullness of the chest, heart pain or even coma, unconsciousness, phlegm wheezing in the throat, white, slimy tongue fur, and a slippery pulse

Treatment principles: Transform phlegm and open the portals

Guiding formula: *Di Tan Tang*

Medicinals: Rhizoma Pinelliae Ternatae (*Ban Xia*), Rhizoma Praeparatus Cum Fellim Bovim (*Dan Nan Xing*), Pericarpium Citri Erythrocarpae (*Ju Hong*), Fructus Aurantii (*Zhi Ke*), Sclerotium Poriae Cocos (*Fu Ling*), Radix Panacis Ginseng (*Ren Shen*), Rhizoma Acori Graminei (*Chang Pu*), Caulis Bambusae In Taeniis (*Zhu Ru*), Radix Glycyrrhizae (*Gan Cao*), uncooked Rhizoma Zingiberis (*Sheng Jiang*), Pericarpium Citri Reticulatae (*Chen Pi*)

Formula Explanation: Rhizoma Pinelliae Ternatae dries dampness and transforms phlegm, harmonizes the stomach and downbears counterflow. Pericarpium Citri Reticulatae rectifies the qi and dries dampness, thus dispersing phlegm. Rhizoma Praeparatus Cum Fellim Bovim Arisaematis clears and transforms hot phlegm. Radix Panacis Ginseng greatly supplements the source qi, quiets the spirit, and tranquilizes the emotions. Rhizoma Acori Graminei arouses the spirit and opens the portals. Fructus Aurantii lowers the qi and disperses phlegm. Sclerotium Poriae Cocos blandly seeps and fortifies the spleen. Caulis Bambusae In Taeniis clears and transforms hot phlegm, relieves vexation, and stops vomiting. Uncooked Rhizoma Zingiberis and Fructus Zizyphi Jujubae (*Da Zao*) regulate and harmonize the constructive and defensive. And Radix Glycyrrhizae regulates and harmonizes the preceding medicinals.

Selected acupuncture/moxibustion points: *Bai Hui* (GV 20)⊥, *Ren Zhong* (GV 26)⊥, *Feng Long* (St 40)⊥, *Nei Guan* (Per 6)⊥, *Da Ling* (Per 7)⊥, & *Ju Que* (CV 14)⊥

Formula rationale: Draining *Bai Hui* clears the brain and arouses the spirit. Draining *Ren Zhong* opens the portals and arouses the spirit. *Feng Long* transforms phlegm and discharges fire. *Nei Guan* loosens the chest and rectifies the qi, quiets the spirit and tranquilizes the emotions. *Ju Que* is the front *mu* point of the heart. Draining it is able to clear heat and calm the spirit. Draining *Da Ling* eliminates evil and scatters stasis, thus opening the heart portals.

F. *Gan Feng Nei Dong Xing*
Liver Wind Stirring Internally Pattern

Clinical manifestations: Dizziness and distention of the head, severe vertigo, low back and knee soreness and weakness, deviated mouth and eyes, unclear speech, spasms and convulsions, a red tongue with a yellow or white, slimy fur, and a wiry, forceful pulse

Treatment principles: Settle the liver and extinguish wind

Guiding formula: *Zhen Gan Xi Feng Tang Jia Jian*

Medicinals: Os Draconis (*Sheng Long Gu*), Concha Ostreae (*Sheng Mu Li*), Plastrum Testudinis (*Gui Ban*), Radix Achyrantis Bidentatae (*Niu Xi*), Haemititum (*Dai Zhe Shi*), Radix Albus Paeoniae Lactiflorae (*Bai Shao*), Fructus Schizandrae Chinensis (*Wu Wei Zi*), Tuber Asparagi Cochinensis (*Tian Men Dong*), Radix Scrophulariae Ningpoensis (*Yuan Shen*), Herba Artemisiae Capillaris (*Yin Chen*),

Fructus Meliae Toosendan (*Chuan Lian Zi*), stir-fried Fructus Germinatus Hordei Vulgaris (*Chao Mai Ya*), Ramulus Uncariae Cum Uncis (*Gou Teng*), Fructus Gardeniae Jasminoidis (*Zhi Zi*), Concha Haliotidis (*Shi Jue Ming*), Radix Glycyrrhizae (*Gan Cao*)

Formula explanation: Os Draconis and Concha Ostreae level the liver and lie low yang. Haemititum descends the qi and settles counterflow. Radix Achyranthis Bidentatae leads the blood and moves it downward, thus levelling source yang. It also enriches and nourishes the liver and kidneys. Plastrum Testudinis, Radix Achyranthis Bidentatae, Tuber Asparagi Cochinensis, and Radix Albus Paeoniae Lactiflorae enrich yin and nourish fluids in order to restrict or control source yang. Herba Artemisiae Capillaris and Fructus Meliae Toosendan are the main medicinals to clear and discharge the fire of liver yang. Fructus Germinatus Hordei Vulgaris harmonizes the stomach so as to protect the stomach from being damaged by the heavy metal and stone medicinals. Concha Haliotidis levels the liver and lies low yang. Ramulus Uncariae Cum Uncis clears heat and levels the liver, eliminates wind and stops aching, *i.e.*, spasms and convulsions. Fructus Gardeniae Jasminoidis clears heat and descends fire, cools the blood and resolves toxins. The entire formula as a whole settles the liver, extinguishes wind, and stops spasm.

Selected acupuncture/moxibustion points: *Tai Chong* (Liv 3)⊥, *He Gu* (LI 4)⊥, *Bai Hui* (GV 20)⊥, *Fu Liu* (Ki 7)⊤, *Feng Long* (St 40)⊥, & *Xing Jian* (Liv 2)⊥

Formula rationale: Draining *Ba Hui* extinguishes wind and lies low yang, expels wind and scatters evil, frees the flow of the channels and resolves pain. Draining *Xing Jian* extinguishes wind and lies low yang, clears and discharges liver fire. Supplementing *Fu Liu* enriches kidney water and levels liver yang. Draining *He Gu* clears and discharges heat evils. *Feng Long* transforms phlegm turbidity and drains fire. *Tai Chong* and *He Gu* together bilaterally are known as the "four passes". Draining them courses wind and clears heat, levels the liver and extinguishes wind.

G. *Yin Yang Liang Shuai Xing*
Yin & Yang Dual Debility Pattern

Clinical manifestations: Bodily emaciation, mind or essence spirit withered and fatigued, body warm, limbs chilled, heart palpitations, blurred vision, dizziness, tinnitus, tongue fur pale with scant fluids or no fur, and an extremely fine pulse on the verge of exhaustion or severance.

Treatment principles: Boost the qi and nourish the blood, enrich yin and recover the pulse

Guiding formula: *Zhi Gan Cao Tang*

Medicinals: Mix-fried Radix Glycyrrhizae (*Zhi Gan Cao*), Radix Panacis Ginseng (*Ren Shen*), Prepared Radix Rehmanniae (*Shu Di*), Cortex Cinnamomi (*Gui Pi*), Gelatinum Corii Asini (*E Jiao*), Tuber Ophiopogonis Japonicae (*Mai Dong*), uncooked Rhizoma Zingiberis (*Sheng Jiang*), Fructus Zizyphi Jujubae (*Da Zao*)

Formula explanation: Mix-fried Radix Glycyrrhizae, sweet and warm, boosts the qi, relaxes urgency, and nourishes the heart. Radix Panacis Ginseng greatly supplements the source qi. Tuber Ophiopogonis Japonicae nourishes yin and engenders fluids. Prepared Radix Rehmanniae and Gelatinum Corii Asini enrich yin and nourish the blood. Adding some Cortex Cinnamomi warms the yang and frees the flow of the vessels, hence normalizing the circulation of blood and fluids. Uncooked Rhizoma Zingiberis and Fructus Zizyphi Jujubae regulate and harmonize the constructive and defensive. These medicinals together boost the qi and nourish the blood, enrich yin and recover the pulse.

If the flesh and muscles are shrivelled and shrunken, and if there are a dry mouth and lips, deep-set eyes, vexation and agitation or coma, shortness of breath, and facial color tidally red, all symptoms of perishing yin, one should use *Sheng Mai San* to enrich yin and increase fluids, boost the qi and restrain yin.

If there is great sweating, dribbling and dripping, counterflow chilling of the four extremities, a pale white facial complexion, weak, tiny respiration, and a minute, exhausted pulse, all symptoms of perishing yang, one should use *Shen Fu Tang* to boost the qi, return yang, and secure desertion.

Selected acupuncture/moxibustion points: *Guan Yuan* (CV 4)ᴀ, *Qi Hai* (CV 6)ᴀ, *Bai Hui* (GV 20)ᴀ, *San Yin Jiao* (Sp 6)ᴛ, & *Nei Guan* (Per 6)|

Formula rationale: Needling followed by moxibustion at *Guan Yuan* can greatly supplement the source qi. *Qi Hai* supplements the middle and boosts the qi. Together these two points bank and supplement both pre and postnatal roots and secure the lower source. Moxaing *Bai Hui* upbears the yang and boosts the qi. *San Yin Jiao* enriches yin and nourishes the blood. Even supplementation and drainage of *Nei Guan* empowers the heart and quiets the spirit, boosts the qi and loosens the chest, and sends out the blood and recovers the pulse.

For those with severe sweating which will not stop, add *Yin Xi* (Ht 6) to enrich yin and restrain sweating. For perishing of yin or perishing yang manifesting as desertion, *i.e.*, fainting or loss of consciousness, *Ren Zhong* (GV 26) with draining method arouses the brain and opens the portals. Moxaing *Guan Yuan* (CV 4) and *Shen Que* (CV 8) returns yang and secures desertion.

AIDS is a systemic disease which affects the entire body. All the viscera become involved in this disease. The above patterns do not categorically cover all clinically encountered patterns, nor can they. Neither do these patterns necessarily change in a fixed course. A patient may present different patterns at different stages or complications of many patterns simultaneously. Therefore, in clinical practice, treatment based on *bian zheng* or the discrimination of patterns requires a very high degree of acumen when it comes to actual cases.

When treating AIDS with acupuncture/moxibustion, the sterilization of the needles before and after each needling should be greatly emphasized or one should use disposable needles to prevent infection of both doctors and other patients.

5

Ai Zi Bing Zhu Zheng De Bian Zheng Zhi Liao

The *Bian Zheng* Treatment of AIDS' Main Pathoconditions

There are a large number of clinical manifestations one may encounter in the course of AIDS. However, in any individual patient, only one or a few pathological conditions tend to manifest (at any given time) depending upon the individual and the stage of development of their disease. Traditional Chinese Medicine refers to these as the main pathoconditions. Below are the most commonly seen, major pathoconditions and their treatment based on a discrimination of patterns.

I. *Fa Re*
Fever

Fever is one of the common pathoconditions associated with AIDS. Typically there is fever in the ARC stage. This is usually a prolonged, low-grade fever without any clear cause. Its TCM or disease cause is usually quite complicated. In the full blown AIDS stage, due to the body's compromised immune function, there commonly are opportunistic infections. In this stage, fever is usually more than moderate. In addition, when the early stage of AIDS is accompanied by cancer, there may also be a low-grade fever. The growth and necrosis of tumors and/or accompanying infections may also cause more than a medium degree of fever.

A. *Bing Yin Bing Ji*
Disease Causes, Disease Mechanisms

In the AIDS prodromal stage, fever is mostly due to vacuity and weakness of the viscera and bowels and detriment and damage of the qi, blood, yin, and essence with subsequent loss of balance of the body's yin and yang. When pestilential toxic evils invade internally, they injure yin fluids resulting in deficiency and vacuity of yin essence. When yin wanes, yang gets the upper hand. Water cannot control fire, resulting in yin vacuity fever. As said in the *Jing Yue Quan Shu (The Complete Writings of [Zhang] Jing-yue)*:

> Yin vacuity is capable of fever. This is because, when yin is deficient
> and damaged, water cannot control fire.

If spleen qi is deficient and vacuous and middle qi is insufficient, yin fire may arise internally which results in qi vacuity fever. If the spleen is unable to engender blood for a long time, this results in spleen vacuity blood deficiency. When the blood is vacuous, the body is not nourished. Yin and blood become insufficient to restrain yang, thus giving rise to fever.

In the full blown AIDS stage, the viscera and bowels, qi and blood are deficient and damaged. Invasion by external evils may lead to a struggle between righteous and evil. If there is not enough strength to combat evil, damp heat evils intrude internally giving rise to fever. If evil heat reaches the constructive and blood, constructive yin may be scorched, resulting in such symptoms as high fever, vexation, and thirst. (Also) in the latter stage of AIDS, if there is qi stagnation and blood stasis, tumors may arise. Because blood stasis blocks the channels and network vessels, qi and blood become choppy and stagnant and cannot flow freely. Thus blood stasos can result in fever.

B. *Fen Xing Zhi Liao*
Differentiation & Treatment

1. *Yin Xu Fa Re*
Yin Vacuity Fever

Clinical manifestations: Tidal fever in the afternoon, both cheeks flushed red, a feeling of vexatious heat in the five hearts, night sweats, emaciation, heart palpitations, scant sleep, profuse dreaming, dry mouth and throat, stools either dry or diarrhea, scant, yellow urine, a red tongue with scant fur, and a fine, rapid pulse

Treatment principles: Enrich yin and clear heat

Guiding formula: *Qing Hao Bie Jia Tang*

Medicinals: Radix Stellariae Dichotomae (*Yin Chai Hu*), Cortex Radicis Lycii Chinensis (*Di Gu Pi*), Rhizoma Picrorrhizae (*Hu Huang Lian*), Rhizoma Anemarrhenae (*Zhi Mu*), Herba Artemesiae Apiaceae (*Qing Hao*), Carapax Amydae Sinensis (*Bie Jia*), uncooked Radix Rehmanniae (*Sheng Di*), Radix Glycyrrhizae (*Gan Cao*)

Formula explanation: Carapax Amydae Sinensis, salty and cold, enriches yin. It can cause vacuous heat to recede. Herba Artemisiae Apiaceae, fragrant and aromatic, clears heat and penetrates the network vessels in order to lead evil out to the exterior. Radix Stellariae Dichotomae and Cortex Radicis Lycii Chinensis cool the blood, recede steaming, and clear vacuous heat. Rhizoma Picrorrhizae clears vacuous heat and also clear heat and disinhibits dampness. Uncooked Radix Rehmanniae and Rhizoma Anemarrhenae boost yin and clear heat, and assist Carapax Amydae Sinensis to recede vacuous heat. Cortex Radicis

Moutan clears heat and cools the blood. And Radix Glycyrrhizae rectifies and harmonizes the preceding medicinals.

Selected acupuncture/moxibustion points: *Jian Shi* (Per 5)⊥, *Tai Xi* (Ki 3)⊤, *Da Zhui* (GV 14)|, *Tai Chong* (Liv 3)⊥, & *Qu Chi* (LI 11)⊤

Formula rationale: *Da Zhui* is the meeting point of the hand and foot three yang channels and the *du mai*. *Qu Chi* is the hand *yang ming* sea point. These two points used together are effective for clearing heat. *Jian Shi* is a pericardium channel point. Combined with *Tai Xi*, it has the power to enrich yin and clear heat. *Tai Chong* is the source point of the liver channel. Draining it levels the liver, lies low yang, and downbears vacuous fire.

2. *Qi Xu Fa Re*
   ## Qi Vacuity Fever

Clinical manifestations: Low fever, spontaneous perspiration, emaciation, fatigue, inability to work, lack of strength, a somber white facial complexion, heart palpitations, shortness of breath, disinclination to speak, diminished appetite, loose stools, a pale tongue, and a deep, fine pulse

Treatment principles: Eliminate heat with sweet, warm medicinals

Guiding formula: *Bu Zhong Yi Qi Tang*

Medicinals: Radix Astragali Membranacei (*Huang Qi*), Radix Codonopsis Pilosulae (*Dang Shen*), Rhizoma Atractylodis Macrocephalae (*Bai Zhu*), Radix Angelicae Sinensis (*Dang Gui*), Pericarpium Citri Reticulatae (*Chen Pi*), Rhizoma Cimicifugae (*Sheng Ma*), Radix Bupleuri (*Chai Hu*), mix-fried Radix Glycyrrhizae (*Zhi Gan Cao*)

Formula explanation: Radix Astragali Membranacei is the ruling or main medicinal. It boosts the qi and upbears yang, boosts the defensive and secures the exterior. This is aided by Radix Codonopsis Pilosulae and Rhizoma Atractylodis Macrocephalae which boost the qi and fortify the spleen. Together with the ruling medicinal, these supplement the middle and boost the qi. Pericarpium Citri Reticulatae fortifies the spleen and dries dampness. Radix Angelicae Sinensis nourishes the blood. Adding a little Rhizoma Cimicifugae and Radix Bupleuri aids the main medicinal to boost the qi and upbear yang. Radix Glycyrrhizae rectifies and harmonizes the middle and boosts the qi. All the above medicinals when used together supplement the middle and boost the qi. When central qi is sufficient, fever is spontaneously eliminated.

Selected acupuncture/moxibustion points: *Da Zhui* (GV 14)|, *Qi Hai* (CV 6)▵, *Zu San Li* (St 36)⊤, *Bai Hui* (GV 20)⊤x, & *Zhong Wan* (CV 12)▵

Formula rationale: Even supplementation and drainage of *Da Zhui* clears heat. *Qi Hai* and *Zhong Wan* when used together with supplementing method and then moxaed supplement the center and boost the qi, harmonize the stomach, fortify the spleen, and aid transportation. Needling *Bai Hui* and then moxaing it boosts the qi and upbears yang. *Zu San Li* is the sea point of the *yang ming*. Supplementing it fortifies the spleen and nourishes the stomach, supplements the center and boosts the qi.

3. *Shi Re Yun Jie*
Damp Heat Accumulating & Binding

Clinical manifestations: Fever sometimes high, sometimes low, simultaneously there is headache, heart vexation, fullness of the chest, nausea and even vomiting, edema of the body and limbs, dry mouth, short, red urine, sores on the skin or mouth sores, or diarrhea, yellow, slimy tongue fur, and a slippery, rapid pulse

Treatment principles: Clear heat and resolve toxins, disinhibit dampness and transform turbidity

Guiding formula: *Gan Lu Xiao Du Dan Jia Jian*

Medicinals: Radix Scutellariae Baicalensis (*Huang Qin*), Talcum (*Hua Shi*), Herba Artemisiae Capillaris (*Yin Chen*), Caulis Akebiae (*Mu Tong*), Herba Agastachis Seu Pogostemi (*Huo Xiang*), Rhizoma Belamcandae (*She Gan*), Fructus Forsythiae Suspensae (*Lian Qiao*), Rhizoma Acori Graminei (*Shi Chang Pu*), Fructus Amomi Caradmomi (*Bai Kou Ren*)

Formula explanation: Talcum clears heat and disinhibits dampness. Herba Artemisiae Capillaris and Caulis Akebiae clear and disinhibit damp heat and lead dampness out via urination. Radix Scutellariae Baicalensis clears heat and dries dampness. Fructus Forsythiae Suspensae clears heat and resolves toxins. Bulbus Fritillariae Thunbergii (*Bei Mu*), and Rhizoma Belamcandae resolve toxins and disinhibit the throat. Rhizoma Acori Graminei and Fructus Amomi Cardamomi fragrantly and aromatically transform turbidity, move the qi, and arouse the spleen. Herba Menthae Haplocalycis (*Bo He*) is clear, acrid, cool, and scattering and thus clears and disinhibits the head and eyes.

Selected acupuncture/moxibustion points: *Da Zhui* (GV 14)⊥, *Qu Chi* (LI 11)⊥, *Yin Ling Quan* (Sp 9)⊥, *Zu San Li* (St 36)⊥, *Gong Sun* (Sp 4)⊥

Formula rationale: Draining *Da Zhui* and *Qu Chi* clears heat. *Yin Ling Quan* is the sea point of the spleen channel. Draining it clears and disinhibits damp turbidity and promotes the transportation of the spleen/ stomach. *Gong Sun* is the network point of the spleen channel and one of the meeting points of the eight vessels. Draining it clears heat and cools the blood, resolves toxins and expels dampness. Draining *Zu San Li* clears heat and resolves toxins, harmonizes the middle and fortifies the spleen.

4. *Re Ru Ying Xue*
Heat Enters the Constructive & Blood

Clinical manifestations: Fever, mostly high, vexation and agitation, subcutaneous purpuric hemorrhage, dry mouth, disturbed sleep, or hematemesis, epistaxis, blood in the stools, possible occasional coma, delirium, or convulsions, a deep red tongue, and rapid pulse

Treatment principles: Clear the constructive and cool the blood

Guiding formula: *Qing Ying Tang Jia Jian*

Medicinals: Gypsum Fibrosum (*Sheng Shi Gao*), Folium Daqingye (*Da Qing Ye*), Radix Isatidis Seu Baphicacanthi (*Ban Lan Geng*), Uncooked Radix Rehmanniae (*Sheng Di*), Cortex Radicis Moutan (*Dan Pi*), Radix Scrophulariae Ningpoensis (*Yuan Shen*), Herba Lophatheri Gracilis (*Zhu Ye*), Tuber Ophiopogonis Japonicae (*Mai Dong*), Radix Salviae Miltiorrhizae (*Dan Shen*), Cornu Rhinocerotis (*Xi Jiao*), Rhizoma Coptidis Chinensis (*Huang Lian*), Flos Lonicerae Japonicae (*Yin Hua*)

Formula explanation: Cornu Rhinocerotis, salty and cold, clears hot toxins from the constructive aspect. Folium Daqingye, Radix Isatidis Seu Baphicacanthi, and Flos Lonicerae Japonicae clear heat and resolve toxins. Uncooked Radix Rehmanniae, Tuber Ophiopogonis Japonicae, and Radix Scrophulariae Ningpoensis clear heat and nourish yin. Gypsum Fibrosum, sweet and cold, clears heat, relieves vexation, and stops thirst. Cortex Radicis Moutan resolves toxins and cools the blood. Herba Lophatheri Gracilis and Rhizoma Coptidis Chinensis clear heat, calm the spirit, and pass heat outward to the exterior. This is aided by Radix Salviae Miltiorrhizae which clears heat and cools the blood, quickens the blood and scatters stasis.

Selected acupuncture/moxibustion points: *Da Zhui* (GV 14)⊥, *Qu Chi* (LI 11)⊥, the twelve well points ↓, *Jian Shi* (Per 5)↓, & *Wei Zhong* (Bl 40)↓

Formula rationale: Draining *Da Zhui* and *Qu Chi* clears evil heat. *Jian Shi* is the sea point of the pericardium channel and *Wei Zhong* is that of the bladder channel. Bleeding these two points clears heat from the blood, tranquilizes the heart, cools the blood, and resolves toxins.

Bleeding the twelve well points clears heat from the constructive aspect and resuscitates.

5. *Yu Xue Fa Re*
Stagnant Blood Fever

Clinical manifestations: Fever in the afternoon or night, dry mouth but no thirst, concretions and conglomerations, accumulations and gatherings or swellings in other parts of the body, or possibly scaly skin, purplish points or spots on the tongue, and a wiry or fine, wiry pulse

Treatment principles: Quicken the blood and transform stasis

Guiding formula: *Xue Fu Zhu Yu Tang Jia Jian*

Medicinals: Semen Pruni Persicae (*Tao Ren*), Flos Carthami Tinctorii (*Hong Hua*), Radix Rubrus Paeoniae Lactiflorae (*Chi Shao*), Radix Achyranthis Bidenatae (*Niu Xi*), Radix Angelicae Sinensis (*Dang Gui*), Uncooked Radix Rehmanniae (*Sheng Di*), Radix Ligustici Wallichii Chuanxiong (*Chaun Xiong*), Radix Bupleuri (*Chai Hu*), Fructus Immaturus Aurantii (*Zhi Shi*), Cortex Radicis Moutan (*Dan Pi*), Radix Glycyrrhizae (*Gan Cao*)

Formula explanation: Semen Pruni Persicae and Flos Carthami Tinctorii quicken the blood and transform stasis. Radix Bupleuri harmonizes, resolves, and recedes heat. Uncooked Radix Rehmanniae enriches yin and clears heat in order to engender fluids. Radix Rubrus Paeoniae Lactiflorae clears heat, cools the blood, and expels stasis. Radix Angelicae Sinensis supplements and quickens the blood. Radix Ligustici Wallichii quickens the blood and moves the qi. Radix Achyranthis Bidentatae expels stasis and frees the vessels, leads the blood and moves it downward. Cortex Radicis Moutan cools the blood and resolves toxins. Fructus Immaturus Aurantii moves the qi. And Radix Glycyrrhizae rectifies and harmonizes the preceding medicinals. When the above medicinals are ued together, stasis is expelled and heat cleared.

Selected acupuncture/moxibustion points: *San Yin Jiao* (Sp 6)⊥, *Xue Hai* (Sp 10)⊥, *Shan Zhong* (CV 17)|, *Da Zhui* (GV 14)⊥, & *Qu Chi* (LI 11)⊥

Formula rationale: Draining *San Yin Jiao* quickens the blood, expels stasis, and courses the liver. *Xue Hai* affects the blood portion. Draining it moves the blood, expels stasis, and clears heat from the blood aspect. *Shan Zhong* rectifies the qi and loosens the chest. And draining *Da Zhui* and *Qu Chi* clears heat.

II. *Xiao Shu Fa Li*
Emaciation & Lack of Strength

Progressive weight loss and asthenia are early clinical symptoms of the ARC stage. Despite continuous food intake or prolonged extra-gastrointestinal nutrient feeding, there is still weight loss. This consumption is always progressive. A patient's weight may drop 20-40% compared to their original weight. For reasons which remain unknown, this is often accompanied by extreme loss of strength or asthenia. In addition, prolonged low fever, a rise in metabolic rate, poor appetite, and reduced food intake in the early stages lead to nutrient insufficiency with bodily emaciation combined with asthenia. (Further,) opportunistic infections associated with AIDS may affect the digestive tract resulting in prolonged diarrhea, vomiting, and poor appetite. After some time, blood production becomes impaired with chronic, severe anemia or the production of tumors. This may worsen the case, causing extreme emaciation and asthenia or, in other words, malignant cachexia.

A. Disease Causes, Disease Mechanisms

This condition always arises due to pestilential evils consuming the interior with viscera and bowels, qi and blood deficiency and vacuity and insufficient source qi resulting in no transformation and engenderment. Thus the body is not nourished by the blood. This then causes emaciation and lack of strength. The crux of the disease mechanism is deficiency and vacuity of the viscera and bowels. Among the viscera, the spleen and kidneys are the ruling ones. The spleen and stomach are the

99

postnatal root. The spleen governs building, transportation, engenderment, and transformation. The stomach governs reception and digestion. When they function together and transport and transform, the source of qi and blood transformation is sufficient. The body's qi is full and the body is strong. But if the spleen/stomach are deficient and vacuous, the central qi is insufficient. This may lead to dysfunction in receiving food and transportation and transformation. The source of engenderment and transformation of qi and blood and fluids and humors becomes insufficient. Thus the source of transformation lacks a root. Qi and blood are not full. This results in wasting of the flesh and muscles and lack of strength or asthenia. The kidneys are the prenatal root. They store essence and transform qi to fill the form. If the kidneys are vacuous, the root is deficient and lacking. With nothing to nourish essence and fill the form, this condition arises.

B. Differentiation & Treatment

1. *Pi Wei Qi Xu*
Spleen/Stomach Qi Vacuity

Clinical manifestations: Emaciation, lassitude of the spirit, lack of strength, no desire for food or drink, abdominal distention after eating, loose, flimsy stools or diarrhea, shortness of breath, disinclination to speak, a sallow, yellow complexion, a pale tongue with white fur, and an vacuous, weak pulse

Treatment principles: Fortify the spleen and boost the qi

Guiding formula: *Si Jun Zi Tang Jia Wei*

Medicinals: Radix Panacis Ginseng (*Ren Shen*), Rhizoma Atractylodis Macrocephalae (*Bai Zhu*), Sclerotium Poriae Cocos (*Fu Ling*), Radix Astragali Membranacei (*Huang Qi*), Radix Dioscoreae Oppositae (*Shan Yao*), Rhizoma Pinelliae Ternatae (*Ban Xia*), Fructus Amomi (*Sha Ren*), Radix Auklandiae (*Mu Xiang*), Pericarpium Citri Reticulatae (*Chen Pi*), mix-fried Radix Glycyrrhizae (*Zhi Gan Cao*)

Formula explanation: Radix Panacis Ginseng supplements the spleen, boosts the qi, and greatly supplements the source qi. Rhizoma Atractylodis Macrocephalae fortifies the spleen and dries dampness. Sclerotium Poriae Cocos seeps dampness and fortifies the spleen. Radix Astragali Membranacei used together with Radix Panacis Ginseng supplement the strength or power of the qi. Radix Dioscoreae Oppositae boosts the qi and supplements the spleen. Rhizoma Pinelliae Ternatae and Pericarpium Citri Reticulatae both dry dampness and fortify the spleen. Fructus Amomi and Radix Auklandiae fortify the spleen and rectify the qi in order to assist transportation and transformation. And mix-fried Radix Glycyrrhizae, sweet as it is, relaxes and harmonizes the middle.

Selected acupuncture/moxibustion points: *Pi Shu* (Bl 20)т, *Wei Shu* (Bl 21)т, *Zhong Wan* (CV 12)т, *Zu San Li* (St 36)т, & *Guan Yuan* (CV 4)▵

Formula rationale: *Pi Shu* and *Wei Shu* are both back *shu* points. Supplementing them fortifies the spleen and boosts the qi, harmonizes the center and disperses conduction. Supplementing *Zhong Wan* fortifies the stomach qi and supplements the center. *Zu San Li* is the sea point of the *yang ming* channel. It supplements and boosts the postnatal root. Needling and then adding moxibustion at *Guan Yuan* supplements and boosts the prenatal, supplements the source of essence, and thus fills the form.

2. *Qi Xue Xu Ruo*
Qi & Blood Vacuity & Weakness

Clinical manifestations: Fatigue, inability to work, lack of strength, emaciation, a lustreless facial complexion, dizziness, blurred vision, shortness of breath, heart palpitations, lack of sleep, no desire for food or drink, a pale tongue, and a fine, weak or vacuous, forceless pulse

Treatment principles: Boost the qi and nourish the blood

Guiding formula: *Ba Zhen Tang Jia Wei*

101

Medicinals: Radix Codonopsis Pilosulae (*Dang Shen*), Rhizoma Atractylodis Macrocephalae (*Bai Zhu*), Radix Astragali Membranacei (*Huang Qi*), Sclerotium Poriae Cocos (*Fu Ling*), Radix Angelicae Sinensis (*Dang Gui*), Prepared Radix Rehmanniae (*Shu Di*), Radix Ligustici Wallichii (*Chuan Xiong*), Radix Albus Paeoniae Lactiflorae (*Bai Shao*), Gelatinum Corii Asini (*E Jiao*), mix-fried Radix Glycyrrhizae (*Zhi Gan Cao*)

Formula explanation: Radix Codonopsis Pilosulae and Prepared Radix Rehmanniae boost the qi and nourish the blood. Sclerotium Poriae Cocos and Rhizoma Atractylodis Macrocephalae fortify the spleen and dry dampness. Radix Angelicae Sinensis supplements and quickens the blood. Radix Albus Paeoniae Lactiflorae nourishes the blood and harmonizes the constructive. Gelatinum Corii Asini supplements the blood and enriches the moist. Adding a little Radix Ligustici Wallichii quickens the blood and moves the qi. And mix-fried Radix Glycyrrhizae rectifies and harmonizes the preceding medicinals.

Selected acupuncture/moxibustion points: *Zu San Li* (St 36)⊤, *Guan Yuan* (CV 4)⊤, *Pi Shu* (Bl 20)⊤, *Xue Hai* (Sp 10)⊤, & *Ge Shu* (Bl 17)⊤

Formula rationale: *Zu San Li* supplements and boosts the postnatal, fortifies the spleen and aids transportation. Needling *Guan Yuan* and then moxaing it supplements the prenatal essence. *Pi Shu* fortifies the spleen and aids transportation. *Xue Hai* nourishes and quickens the blood. *Ge Shu* is the reunion point of the blood. Supplementing it can nourish yin blood, rectifies the blood, and quickens the blood as well as stops bleeding. When these points are used together, the growth of qi and blood is obtained and thus the form is spontaneously filled.

3. *Fei Yin Bu Zu*
Lung Yin Insufficiency

Clinical manifestations: Emaciation, lassitude of the spirit, lack of strength, dry cough with scant phlegm, dry mouth and throat, tidal fever, night sweats, vexatious heat in the five centers, a red tongue with scant fluids, and a fine, rapid pulse

Treatment principles: Nourish yin and clear the lungs

Guiding formula: *Bai He Gu Jin Tang Jia Jian*

Medicinals: Prepared Radix Rehmanniae (*Shu Di*), Uncooked Radix Rehmanniae (*Sheng Di*), Bulbus Lilii (*Bai He*), Tuber Ophiopogonis Japonicae (*Mai Dong*), Bulbus Fritillariae Thunbergii (*Bei Mu*), Radix Angelicae Sinensis (*Dang Gui*), Radix Albus Paeoniae Lactiflorae (*Bai Shao*), Radix Scrophulariae Ningpoensis (*Yuan Shen*), Radix Platycodi Grandiflori (*Jie Geng*), Radix Glycyrrhizae (*Gan Cao*)

Formula explanation: In this formula, Uncooked Radix Rehmanniae clears heat and engenders fluids. Bulbus Lilii and Prepared Radix Rehmanniae enrich and nourish the lungs and kidneys. Tuber Ophiopogonis Japonicae aids Bulbus Lilii in moistening the lungs and stopping cough. Bulbus Fritillariae Thunbergii moistens the lungs, transforms phlegm, and stops cough. Radix Scrophulariae Ningpoensis enriches yin and clears heat. Radix Angelicae Sinensis and Radix Albus Paeoniae Lactiflorae enrich yin and supplement the blood. Adding a little Radix Platycodi Grandiflori disinhibits the throat and expels phlegm. Radix Glycyrrhizae rectifies the foregoing medicinals.

Selected acupuncture/moxibustion points: *Fei Shu* (Bl 13)⊤, *Gao Huang* (Bl 43)⊤, *Chi Ze* (Lu 5)⊥, *Zhong Fu* (Lu 1)⊥, & *Tai Yuan* (Lu 9)⊤

Formula rationale: In this formula, *Fei Shu* and *Zhong Fu* are used together as *shu* and *mu* points to supplement the lungs and nourish yin. *Gao Huang* is a main point for supplementing vacuous taxation. Supplementing it fills and boosts the physical form. *Chi Ze* is the lung channel sea point. Draining it nourishes yin, clears heat, and stops coughing. *Tai Yuan* is the source point of the lungs. It can supplement vacuity in the lung organ.

4. *Shen Yin Kui Xu*
Kidney Yin Deficient & Vacuous

Clinical manifestations: Emaciation, exhaustion and lack of strength, low back and knee soreness and weakness, tinnitus, vexatious heat in the five hearts, disturbed sleep, night sweats, seminal emission, a red tongue with scant fur, and a fine, rapid pulse

Treatment principles: Enrich and supplement kidney yin

Guiding formula: *Da Bu Yin Wan Jia Wei*

Medicinals: Prepared Radix Rehmanniae (*Shu Di*), Rhizoma Anemarrhenae (*Zhi Mu*), Cortex Phellodendri (*Huang Bai*), Plastrum Testudinis (*Gui Ban*), Gelatinum Corii Asini (*E Jiao*), Radix Dioscoreae Oppositae (*Shan Yao*), Fructus Corni Officinalis (*Shan Zhu Yu*), Sclerotium Poriae Cocos (*Fu Ling*), Cortex Radicis Moutan (*Dan Pi*), Rhizoma Alismatis (*Ze Xie*)

Formula explanation: Prepared Radix Rehmanniae enriches and supplements kidney yin. Plastrum Testudinis enriches yin and lies low yang in order to recede vacuous heat. Cortex Phellodendri and Rhizoma Anemarrhenae clear and discharge ministerial fire, thus enrich yin and clear heat, fill the essence and nourish yin. Gelatinum Corii Asini enriches yin and nourishes the blood. Radix Dioscoreae Oppositae fortifies the spleen and boosts the qi. Fructus Corni Officinalis enriches and nourishes the liver and kidneys. Sclerotium Poriae Cocos blandly seeps, thus clearing heat. Cortex Radicis Moutan discharges fire and cools the blood. Rhizoma Alismatis clears and drains kidney fire. When all these medicinals are used together, true yin is nourished, vacuous fire is cleared internally, and the condition is automatically relieved.

Selected acupuncture/moxibustion points: *Shen Shu* (Bl 23)⟙, *San Yin Jiao* (Sp 6)⟙, *Tai Xi* (Ki 3)⟙, *Shen Men* (Ht 7)⟂, *Zhi Shi* (Bl 52)⟙, & *Zu San Li* (St 36)⟙

Formula rationale: *Shen Shu* enriches and supplements kidney yin. *San Yin Jiao* is the meeting point of the three foot yin. It can enrich and supplement yin, thus help regulate yin and yang. *Tai Xi* enriches and supplements the kidneys which are the source of yin and yang. *Zu San Li* boosts the qi and fortifies the spleen, promotes qi and blood engenderment and transformation. *Shen Men* is the source point of the heart channel. Draining it tranquilizes the heart and quiets the spirit, thus automatically calming sleep. *Zhi Shi* supplements the kidneys and boosts the qi, therefore sealing the treasury of the essence chamber.

III. *Fu Xie* Diarrhea

AIDS patients very frequently suffer from diarrhea where their stools are like water. Usually this is not so serious in the ARC stage. But as ARC develops into full blown AIDS, there are an increasing number of infections, and these infections may result in death. The causes of diarrhea in many patients are not entirely clear. In some patients, specific infectious microbes can be found, such as *Bacillus dysenterica, Salmonella, Vibrio jejuni, Cryptosporidia,* Cytomegalovirus, etc. However, in other patients, no clear(-cut) etiological factors can be found. Among these patients, perhaps, various infections have become chronic, thus causing vacuous desertion diarrhea.

A. Disease Causes, Disease Mechanisms

In TCM, this pathocondition is classified as *xie xie* or diarrhea. This condition's cause is mostly due to righteous qi internally vacuous and invasion by external evils. AIDS' evil, pestilential toxins may damage and injure the spleen and stomach as well as the large and small intestines. This, in turn, causes viscera and bowels vacuity and weakness and susceptibility to invasion by external evils. The spleen governs transportation and transformation and the stomach governs reception and digestion. When pestilential evils damage and injure these, the spleen/stomach become vacuous and weak. They become unable to receive water and grains and to transport and transform nutrient essence. Water and grains accumulate internally and clear and turbid are not separated. Both are passed down together resulting in diarrhea. In full blown AIDS, the viscera and bowels are deficient and vacuous and the function of the spleen/stomach is vacuous and weak. This results in cold damp and damp heat evils invading internally. This may lead to further dysfunction of the spleen and stomach resulting in diarrhea. In addition, long-standing AIDS may cause vacuity of kidney yang. Insufficient yang qi cannot warm. This may also lead to the spleen not transporting and transforming and thus result in diarrhea. In this situation, diarrhea is always more serious.

B. Differentiation & Treatment

1. *Han Shi Zu Zhi*
Cold Dampness Obstructing & Stagnating

Clinical manifestations: Diarrhea clear and watery, abdominal distention and borborygmus accompanied by fullness in the chest, vomiting, no desire for food or drink, physical exhaustion, lack of strength, thirst but not drinking much, no or slight fever, limbs and body sore and painful, white, slimy tongue fur, and a slippery pulse

Treatment principles: Fragrantly and aromatically transform turbidity, disinhibit dampness, and transport the spleen

Guiding formula: *Huo Xiang Zheng Qi San Jia Jian*

Medicinals: Herba Agastachis Seu Pogostemi (*Huo Xiang*), Sclerotium Poriae Cocos (*Fu Ling*), Rhizoma Alismatis (*Ze Xie*), Rhizoma Atractylodis Macrocephalae (*Bai Zhu*), Massa Medica Fermentata (*Liu Qu*), Fructus Crataegi (*Shan Zha*), Radix Auklandiae (*Mu Xiang*), Fructus Amomi (*Sha Ren*), Cortex Magnoliae Officinalis (*Hou Bu*), Pericarpium Citri Reticulatae (*Chen Pi*), Rhizoma Pinelliae Ternatae (*Ban Xia*), Pericarpium Arecae Catechu (*Da Fu Pi*), Fructus Zizyphi Jujubae (*Da Zao*), Radix Glycyrrhizae (*Gan Cao*)

Formula explanation: Herba Agastachis Seu Pogostemi fragrantly and aromatically transforms turbidity, harmonizes the stomach, and wakes the spleen. Rhizoma Pinelliae Ternatae dries dampness and downbears the qi, harmonizes the stomach and stops vomiting. Cortex Magnoliae Officinalis and Pericarpium Arecae Catechu move the qi and transform dampness. Sclerotium Poriae Cocos and Rhizoma Atractylodis Macrocephalae fortify the spleen and transport dampness. Pericarpium Citri Reticulatae rectifies the qi and dries dampness. Radix Platycodi Grandiflori (*Jie Geng*) leads and smooth the qi mechanism. Radix Auklandiae and Fructus Amomi transport the spleen and transform dampness, rectify the qi and stop pain. Fructus Crataegi and Massa Medica Fermentata disperse food and lead off stagnation. Rhizoma Alismatis seeps and disinhibits damp evils. Radix Glycyrrhizae and Fructus Zizyphi Jujubae fortify the spleen and harmonize the stomach, transform dampness and regulate the middle.

Selected acupuncture/moxibustion points: *Tian Shu* (St 25)⊥, *He Gu* (LI 4)⊥, *Yin Ling Quan* (Sp 9)⊥, *Zu San Li* (St 36)⊤, & *Zhong Wan* (CV 12)⊤▵

Formula rationale: *Tian Shu* is the front *mu* point of the large intestine. Draining it frees the intestines and leads off stagnation, clears heat and stops diarrhea. *He Gu* transforms dampness and relieves the exterior. *Yin Ling Quan* transports the spleen and transforms dampness. Supplementing *Zu San Li* results in supplementing the spleen and aiding transportation, rectifies and harmonizes the function of the stomach and intestines. Needling and then moxaing *Zhong Wan* warms the spleen and transports dampness, harmonizes the middle and fortifies the stomach.

2. *Shi Re Nei Yun*
Damp Heat Internally Accumulating

Clinical manifestations: Diarrhea with yellow, hot, loose, fetid stools accompanied by fever, vexation and agitation, thirst, abdominal pain, loss of appetite, a burning sensation in the anus, short, yellow urine, yellow, slimy tongue fur, and a slippery, rapid pulse

Treatment principles: Clear heat and disinhibit dampness

Guiding formula: *Ge Gen Qin Lian Tang* plus *Liu Yi San Jia Wei*

Medicinals: Radix Scutellariae Baicalensis (*Huang Qin*), Rhizoma Coptidis Chinensis (*Huang Lian*), Radix Puerariae (*Ge Geng*), Talcum (*Hua Shi*), Sclerotium Poriae Cocos (*Fu Ling*), Rhizoma Alismatis (*Ze Xie*), Semen Plantaginis (*Che Qian Zi*), Fructus Fosythiae Suspensae (*Lian Qiao*), Flos Lonicerae Japonicae (*Yin Hua*), Radix Glycyrrhizae (*Gan Cao*)

Formula explanation: Radix Puerariae clears heat and relieves the exterior as well as upbears yang and stops diarrhea. This is combined with Rhizoma Coptidis Chinensis and Radix Scutellariae Baicalensis which are both bitter and cold and clear and disinhibit stomach/intestinal damp heat. Adding Fructus Forsythiae Suspensae and Flos Lonicerae Japonicae aids the preceding medicinals' ability to clear heat and resolve toxins. Talcum clears heat and disinhibits dampness. Sclerotium Poriae Cocos, Rhizoma Alismatis, and Semen Plantaginis clear and disinhibit damp heat and strengthen the preceding medicinals' ability to disinhibit dampness, cause damp heat to be separated and dispersed, and therefore stop diarrhea. Radix Glycyrrhizae rectifies and harmonizes the preceding medicinals.

Selected acupuncture/moxibustion points: *Tian Shu* (ST 25)⊥, *Qu Chi* (LI 11)⊥, *Shang Ju Xu* (St 37)⊥, & *Yang Ling Quan* (Sp 9)⊥

Formula rationale: Draining *Tian Shu* clears heat and disinhibits dampness, frees the intestines and stops diarrhea. *Qu Chi* clears heat evils. *Shang Ju Xu* is the lower sea point of the large intestine. Draining it clears and disinhibits stomach/intestinal damp heat, rectifies and harmonizes the spleen and stomach, thus automatically stopping diarrhea. Draining *Yin Ling Quan* clears heat and disinhibits dampness.

3. *Pi Wei Xu Ruo*
Spleen/Stomach Vacuity & Weakness

Clinical manifestations: Loose stool with undigested food, emaciation, lassitude of the spirit, lack of strength, diminished appetite, chest fullness and discomfort, a sallow yellow facial complexion, a pale tongue with white fur, and thin, weak pulse

Treatment principles: Fortify the spleen and harmonize the stomach, boost the qi and promote transportation

Guiding formula: *Shen Ling Bai Zhu San Jia Jian*

Medicinals: Radix Codonopsis Pilosulae (*Dang Shen*), Rhizoma Atractylodis Macrocephalae (*Bai Zhu*), Sclerotium Poriae Cocos (*Fu Ling*), Radix Glycyrrhizae (*Gan Cao*), Radix Dioscoreae Oppositae (*Shan Yao*), Semen Nelumbinis Nuciferae (*Lian Rou*), Semen Coicis Lachryma-jobi (*Yi Ren*), Semen Dolichoris (*Bian Dou*), Pericarpium Citri Reticulatae (*Chen Pi*), Fructus Amomi (*Sha Ren*), Radix Auklandiae (*Mu Xiang*)

Formula explanation: In this formula, the ingredients of *Si Jun Zi Tang* boost the qi and fortify the spleen, supplement the center and boost the qi. Sclerotium Poriae Cocos, Semen Coicis Lachryma-jobi, and Semen Dolichoris fortify the spleen and transform dampness. Radix Dioscoreae Oppositae and Semen Nelumbinis Nuciferae fortify the spleen and harmonize the stomach in order to stop diarrhea. Radix Saussureae Seu Vladmiriae and Fructus Amomi harmonize the stomach and wake the spleen, move the qi and loosen the chest. Pericarpium Citri Reticulatae fortifies the spleen, dries dampness, and promotes transportation. Adding a little Radix Platycodi Grandiflori (*Jie Geng*) rectifies and smooths the qi mechanism. And Radix Glycyrrhizae boosts the qi, harmonizes the middle, and rectifies and harmonizes the preceding medicinals.

Selected acupuncture/moxibustion points: *Pi Shu* (Bl 20)⊤, *Zhong Wan* (CV 12)⊤, *Zu San Li* (St 36)⊤, *San Yin Jiao* (Sp 6)⊤ & *Tian Shu* (St 25)|

Formula rationale: *Pi Shu* is the back *shu* point of the spleen. Supplementing it fortifies the spleen and promotes transportation. Needling *Zhong Wan* fortifies the spleen, harmonizes the stomach, and stops vomiting. *Zu San Li* supplements the center and boosts the qi. Supplementing *San Yin Jiao* fortifies the spleen and engenders blood. Even supplementation and drainage of *Tian Shu* disinhibits dampness, frees the intestines, stops diarrhea, and rectifies the function of the spleen and stomach.

4. Shen Yang Xu Shuai
Kidney Yang Vacuity & Debility

Clinical manifestations: Chronic diarrhea which will not stop, feces clear and thin or watery, slight abdominal pain, low back and knee soreness and weakness, body cold, limbs chilled, a somber white facial complexion, mind fading, a pale white tongue with white fur, and a deep, fine pulse

Treatment principles: Supplement the spleen and warm the kidneys, secure, astringe, and stop diarrhea

Guiding formula: *Fu Zi Li Zhong Wan Jia Wei*

Medicinals: Radix Lateralis Praeparatus Aconiti Carmichaeli (*Fu Zi*), Radix Codonopsis Pilosulae (*Dang Shen*), Rhizoma Atractylodis Macrocephalae (*Bai Zhu*), Sclerotium Poriae Cocos (*Fu Ling*), Radix Astragali Membranacei (*Huang Qi*), Fructus Psoraleae Corylifoliae (*Bu Gu Zhi*), Fructus Schizandrae Chinensis (*Wu Wei Zi*), Fructus Terminaliae Chebulae (*He Zi*), dry Rhizoma Zingiberis (*Gan Jiang*), Fructus Myristicae Fragrantis (*Rou Dou Kou*), Radix Glycyrrhizae (*Gan Cao*)

Formula explanation: Radix Lateratis Praeparatus Aconiti Carmichaeli warms and supplements kidney yang. Radix Codonopsis Pilosulae fortifies the spleen, supplements the center, and boosts the qi. Dry Rhizoma Zingiberis rectifies the center and supports yang. Rhizoma Atractylodis Macrocephalae fortifies the spleen and dries dampness. Fructus Psoraleae Corylifoliae warms the kidneys and assists yang. Fructus Myristicae Fragrantis warms the spleen and scatters cold. Adding Radix Astragali Membranacei supplements the qi and lifts prolapse. Sclerotium Poriae Cocos blandly seeps, fortifies the spleen, and disinhibits dampness. Fructus Schizandrae Chinensis and Fructus Terminaliae Chebulae secure, astringe, and stop diarrhea. Radix Glycyrrhizae supplements the center and supports the righteous, rectifies and harmonizes the preceding medicinals.

Selected acupuncture/moxibustion points: *Zu San Li* (St 36)т▵, *Shen Que* (CV 8)▵, *Tian Shu* (St 25)т, *Zhong Wan* (CV 12)т, & *Ming Men* (GV 4)▵

Formula rationale: Supplementing *Zu San Li* boosts the qi and fortifies the spleen. Needling and then moxaing it warms and transports spleen yang. Moxaing *Shen Que* motivates central yang and warms and scatters cold evils. Moxaing *Ming Men* warms and supplements kidney yang. Supplementing *Tian Shu* and *Zhong Wan* fortifies the stomach and harmonizes the middle, rectifies the function of the stomach and intestines.

IV. *Shi Yu Bu Zhen*
Loss of Appetite (Literally, Eating & Drinking Without Gusto)

Poor appetite is also one of the most commonly heard complaints among those suffering from AIDS. Diminished appetite is typically a chronic complaint accompanied by distention and lack of openness and unfoldment in the epigastrium. In the early stage, it is commonly accompanied by fever, night sweats, and weight loss. In addition, emotional depression and bad moods may affect the patient's appetite for food and drink. In the latter stages, various opportunistic infections and the arisal of tumors or cancers may also cause reduction of appetite and loss of taste. Because of stomach and intestinal tract dysfunction, there may be accumulation of qi in the stomach and intestines, and hence there may be abdominal distention, fullness, a lack of ease or unfoldment, and belching.

A. Disease Causes, Disease Mechanisms

Yan shi or "boredom with food" was also called in ancient times *bu si shi* or "not thinking about food", *bu shi shi*, "not liking food", *bu ji bu na*, "not hungry, not accepting", etc. In the *Ling Shu: Mai Du (Spiritual Axis: Vessel Measurements)* it says:

> Spleen qi connects with the mouth. When the spleen is harmonious,
> the mouth can unite with the five grains.

According to this theory, this pathocondition is commonly caused by dysfunction of the spleen/stomach. The spleen and stomach are the organs of reception and storage of food. When viscera and bowel function is damaged and suffers detriment, the spleen/stomach are not able to promote transportation, thus not expelling what has been received. The liver controls coursing and discharge. Spleen transportation and transformation depends upon the liver's coursing and discharge. Emotional depression and unfavorable changes in mood typically lead to the liver's not coursing and discharging. This may further affect the spleen/stomach's functions of receiving and accepting and transporting and transforming, thus resulting in diminished food intake. The spleen prefers hardness and dryness; while the stomach prefers softness and moisture. In the latter stage of AIDS, yin fluids are deficient and consumed. If stomach fluids are scorched or burnt, stomach yin becomes insufficient. There is then no soaking moisture. Inability to move, receive and accept, or rotten and ripen eventually leads to loss of appetite or anorexia.

B. Differentiation & Treatment

1. *Pi Yun Shi Jian*
Spleen Transportation Loses Its Promotion

Clinical manifestations: A lustreless facial complexion, no thought for food and drink or eating but without taste, eructation, acid regurgitation, abdominal distention, foul stools, bodily emaciation, thick, slimy tongue fur, and a slippery pulse

Treatment principles: Disperse food and transform stagnation, fortify the spleen and assist transportation

Guiding formula: *Bao He Wan Jia Jian*

Medicinals: Rhizoma Atractylodis Macrocephalae (*Bai Zhu*), Sclerotium Poriae Cocos (*Fu Ling*), Massa Medica Fermentata (*Shen Qu*), Fructus Crataegi (*Shan Zha*), Rhizoma Pinelliae Ternatae (*Ban Xia*), Pericarpium Citri Reticulatae (*Chen Pi*), Semen Raphani Sativi (*Lai Fu Zi*), Fructus Forsythiae Suspensae (*Lian Qiao*), Endothelium Corneum Gigeriae Galli (*Ji Nei Jin*), Fructus Germinatus Hordei Vulgaris (*Mai Ya*)

Formula explanation: Rhizoma Atractylodis Macrocephalae and Sclerotium Poriae Cocos dry dampness, fortify the spleen, and aid transportation. Fructus Crataegi disperses food and leads off stagnation. This is aided by Massa Medica Fermentata which disperses food and fortifies the spleen. Rhizoma Pinelliae Ternatae and Pericarpium Citri Reticulatae move the qi and transform stagnation, fortify the spleen and harmonize the stomach. Semen Raphani Sativi disperses food and moves the qi. Adding a little Fructus Fosythiae Suspensae clears heat and scatters nodulation. Fructus Germinatus Hordei Vulgaris and Endothelium Corneum Gigeriae Galli transport the spleen, disperse food, and harmonize the middle.

113

Selected acupuncture/moxibustion points: *Zhong Wan* (CV 12)⊥x, *Tian Shu* (St 25)⊥x, *Qi Hai* (CV 6)⊥, *Li Nei Ting* (M-LE-1)⊥, & *Zu San Li* (St 36)|

Formula rationale: Draining and then moxaing *Zhong Wan* and *Tian Shu* disperses food and leads off stagnation, frees and harmonizes the stomach and intestines, and fortifies the spleen and aids transportation. Draining *Qi Hai* moves the qi and transforms stagnation. *Li Nei Ting* is an empirical point. Draining it treats damage from food, stagnations and accumulations. It disperses food and harmonizes the middle. Even supplementation and drainage of *Zu San Li* fortifies the spleen and harmonizes the stomach.

2. *Pi Wei Xu Ruo*
Spleen/Stomach Vacuous & Weak

Clinical manifestations: No thought for food and drink, distention after eating, lassitude of the spirit, lack of strength, shortness of breath, disinclination to speak, dull abdominal pain, loose stools, a pale tongue with white fur, and a slow, weak pulse

Treatment principles: Fortify the spleen and boost the qi

Guiding formula: *Yi Gong San Jia Jian*

Medicinals: Radix Codonopsis Pilosulae (*Dang Shen*), Rhizoma Atractylodis Macrocephalae (*Bai Zhu*), Sclerotium Poriae Cocos (*Fu Ling*), Radix Glycyrrhizae (*Gan Cao*), Pericarpium Citri Reticulatae (*Chen Pi*), Fructus Amomi (*Sha Ren*), Fructus Crataegi (*Shan Zha*)

Formula explanation: Radix Codonopsis Pilosulae, warm and sweet, supplements the center and boosts the qi. Rhizoma Atractylodis Macrocephalae dries dampness and fortifies the spleen. Sclerotium Poriae Cocos blandly seeps, disinhibits dampness, and fortifies the spleen. Pericarpium Citri Reticulatae dries dampness and moves the qi in order to fortify the spleen. Fructus Amomi transforms dampness, moves the qi, warms the middle, and fortifies the spleen. This is assisted by Fructus Crataegi which disperses food and transforms stagnations/accumulations. Radix Glycyrrhizae is sweet and arouses and harmonizes the middle, rectifies and harmonizes the preceding medicinals.

Selected acupuncture/moxibustion points: *Zu San Li* (St 36)т, *Zhong Wan* (CV 12)т△, *Pi Shu* (Bl 20)т, & *He Gu* (LI 4)т

Formula rationale: Supplementing *Zu San Li* fortifies the spleen and boosts the qi, thus supplementing the postnatal root. Needling and then adding moxa at *Zhong Wan* warms the stomach and harmonizes the middle in order to aid spleen transportation. Supplementing *Pi Shu* boosts the spleen and stomach. And supplementing *He Gu* boosts the qi and secures the exterior, moves the qi and engenders blood. Used together, these points supplement the spleen, boost the qi, and aid the function of transportation. Thus the condition is spontaneously relieved.

3. *Gan Qi Fan Wei*
Liver Qi Invades the Stomach

Clinical manifestations: Loss of appetite, belching and hiccups, emotional depression, chest and lateral costal distention and fullness or distention and pain, a pale tongue with white fur, and a wiry pulse

Treatment principles: Soothe the liver and harmonize the stomach

Guiding formula: *Xiao Yao San Jia Jian*

Medicinals: Radix Angelicae Sinensis (*Dang Gui*), Sclerotium Poriae Cocos (*Fu Ling*), Radix Albus Paeoniae Lactiflorae (*Bai Shao*), Rhizoma Atractylodis Macrocephalae (*Bai Zhu*), Radix Bupleuri (*Chai Hu*), Radix Codonopsis Pilosulae (*Dang Shen*), Radix Auklandiae (*Mu Xiang*), Radix Glycyrrhizae (*Gan Cao*)

Formula explanation: Radix Bupleuri soothes the liver and resolves depression. Radix Albus Paeoniae Lactiflorae and Radix Angleicae Sinensis supplement the blood and harmonize the constructive in order to regulate the liver. Rhizoma Atractylodis Macrocephalae and Sclerotium Poriae Cocos dry dampness and fortify the spleen so as to aid spleen transportation. Adding Radix Codonopsis Pilosulae, sweet and warm, boosts the qi. Radix Auklandiae moves the qi and courses the liver, fortifies the spleen and assists transportation. Radix Glycyrrhizae assists spleen transportation and rectifies and harmonizes the preceding medicinals.

Selected acupuncture/moxibustion points: *Zhong Wan* (CV 12)|, *Zu San Li* (St 36)⊥, *Nei Guan* (Per 6)⊥, *Tai Chong* (Liv 3)⊥, & *Qi Men* (Liv 14)⊥

Formula rationale: Even supplementation and drainage of *Zhong Wan* harmonizes the middle and fortifies the stomach. Draining *Zu San Li* balances and rectifies the stomach and intestines, fortifies the spleen and aids transportation. *Nei Guan* is the network point of the pericardium. Draining it rectifies the qi and broadens the middle, quiets the spirit and relieves vexation. *Tai Chong* is the source point of the liver channel. *Qi Men* is the front *mu* point of the liver channel. Draining these courses the liver and resolves depression.

4. *Wei Yin Bu Zu*
Stomach Yin Insufficiency

Clinical manifestations: No thought of food and drink or hunger with loss of appetite, dry mouth with desire to drink, dry, red lips, stools mostly dry and knotted, short, scant urine, skin dry and lacking lustre, a red tongue usually uncoated and smooth, and a fine, rapid pulse

Treatment principles: Enrich yin and nourish the stomach

Guiding formula: *Yi Wei Tang Jia Wei*

Medicinals: Radix Glehniae Littoralis (*Sha Shen*), Tuber Ophiopogonis Japonicae (*Mai Dong*), Uncooked Radix Rehmanniae (*Sheng Di*), Rhizoma Polygonati Odorati (*Yu Zhu*), Herba Dendrobii (*Shi Hu*), Cortex Radicis Moutan (*Dan Pi*), Radix Trichosanthis Kirlowii (*Tian Hua Fen*), Radix Scrophulariae Ningpoensis (*Yuan Shen*)

Formula explanation: Radix Glehniae Littoralis and Tuber Ophiopogonis Japonicae enrich yin, engender fluids, and boost the stomach. Uncooked Radix Rehmanniae clears heat, engenders fluids, and stops thirst. Rhizoma Polygonati Odorati and Herba Dendrobii nourish the stomach and engender fluids, enrich yin and clear heat. Cortex Radicis Moutan cools the blood and recedes heat. Radix Trichosanthis Kirlowii clears heat and engenders fluids. Used together, these medicinals enrich yin and nourish the stomach. Thus this pathocondition is spontaneously relieved.

Selected acupuncture/moxibustion points: *Zu San Li* (St 36)|, *San Yin Jiao* (Sp 6)⊤, *Fu Liu* (Ki 7)⊤, *Tai Xi* (Ki 3)⊤, & *Tian Shu* (St 25)⊥

Formula rationale: *Zu San Li* is chosen to harmonize the stomach, fortify the spleen, and aid transportation. Supplementing *San Yin Jiao* and *Fu Liu* enriches yin, boosts the stomach, and engenders fluids. Supplementing *Tai Xi* enriches and supplements kidney yin. Draining *Tian Shu* leads off stagnation, balances and regulates the stomach and intestines, and thus automatically regulates the stools. The above points used together enrich yin and nourish the stomach. When yin fluids are sufficient, appetite will grow and this condition will be automatically relieved.

V. *Ou Tu*
Vomiting

Vomiting is another of the commonly seen pathoconditions of AIDS patients. It is usually seen in the ARC stage and is usually accompanied by other symptoms of the digestive tract, such as diarrhea. However, occasionally nausea and vomiting are the main manifestations. Though its etiology is not very clear, (vomiting) is always a very serious condition since it may rapidly cause dehydration and other dangerous pathological changes.

A. Disease Causes, Disease Mechanisms

The stomach governs reception and acceptance and is harmonious when downbearing. If a patient's viscera and bowels, qi and blood are deficient and vacuous, the vacuous stomach will not be harmonious. Qi counterflows upward resulting in vomiting. Its causes must be carefully studied. The first is spleen/stomach root vacuity plus invasion by external evils. Invasion attacks the stomach bowel. This causes the stomach to loose its harmonious descension. Water and grains, *i.e.*, food and liquids, follow qi which counterflows upward and manifests as vomiting. The second cause is spleen/stomach vacuity and weakness causing damage to the middle qi. If the spleen/stomach become unable to accept water and grains, the nutrient essence of water and grains are not able to be transformed and create qi and blood. This may further result in cold dampness accumulating in the middle, (thus causing vomiting). Also, in prolonged cases of AIDS, stomach yin is insufficient, thus losing its moist descension and also resulting in vomiting. As stated in the *Zheng Zhi Hui Bu (A Supplemental Collection of Patterns and Treatments)*:

> When yin vacuity turns into vomiting, not only the stomach is sick.
> What is called *wu yin* or no yin is vomiting.

In addition, when the spleen is vacuous and loses its transportation, water dampness collects inside and transforms into phlegm and fluids. This stagnates/accumulates in the stomach and middle. Fluid evils counterflow upward resulting in vomiting.

B. Differentiation & Treatment

1. *Wai Xie Fan Wei*
External Evils Attack the Stomach

Clinical manifestations: Vomiting, possible fever and fear of cold, chest and epigastric oppression and fullness, nausea, a heavy sensation in the body, headache, white, slimy or thin, yellow tongue fur, and a soggy, relaxed pulse

Treatment principles: Course and scatter external evils, harmonize the middle and transform dampness

Guiding formula: *Huo Xiang Zheng Qi San Jia Jian*

Medicinals: Herba Agastachis Seu Pogostemi (*Huo Xiang*), Folium Perillae Frutescentis (*Zi Su*), Rhizoma Pinelliae Ternatae (*Ban Xia*), Pericarpium Citri Reticulatae (*Chen Pi*), Sclerotium Poriae Cocos (*Fu Ling*), Herba Eupatorii Fortunei (*Pei Lan*), Pericarpium Arecae Catechu (*Da Fu Pi*), Rhizoma Atractylodis Macrocephalae (*Bai Zhu*), Radix Glycyrrhizae (*Gan Cao*), Fructus Zizyphi Jujubae (*Da Zao*)

Formula explanation: Herba Agastachis Seu Pogostemi fragrantly and aromatically transforms turbidity, harmonizes the stomach, and rectifies the spleen. Rhizoma Pinelliae Ternatae dries dampness, harmonizes the stomach, and stops vomiting. Folium Perillae Frutescentis fragrantly and aromatically transforms dampness, exteriorizes and scatters external evils. Pericarpium Citri Reticulatae dries dampness, fortifies the spleen, and moves the qi. Pericarpium Arecae Catechu moves the qi and disinhibits dampness. Sclerotium Poriae Cocos blandly seeps and fortifies the spleen. Rhizoma Atractylodis Macrocephalae fortifies the spleen and dries dampness. Adding Herba Eupatorii Fortunei harmonizes the middle and transforms dampness. Radix Glycyrrhizae and Fructus Zizyphi Jujubae regulate and harmonize the spleen and stomach.

Selected acupuncture/moxibustion points: *Nei Guan* (Per 6)⊥, *Zhong Wan* (CV 12)⊥, *Zu San Li* (St 36)⊥, & *He Gu* (LI 4)⊥

Formula rationale: *Nei Guan*, one of the meeting points of the eight vessels, is chosen to rectify the qi, harmonize the stomach, and stop vomiting. Draining *Zhong Wan* loosens the chest and rectifies the qi, fortifies the spleen and transforms dampness. *Zu San Li* balances and rectifies the function of the stomach and intestines, fortifies the spleen and moves the qi. Draining *He Gu* courses the exterior and scatters evils.

2. *Pi Wei Xu Han*
Spleen/Stomach Vacuous Cold

Clinical manifestations: Frequent vomiting accompanied by diarrhea in prolonged cases, a somber white facial complexion, mind exhausted and weary, four limbs not warm, a pale tongue with white fur, and a fine, forceless pulse

Treatment principles: Warm the middle and fortify the spleen, harmonize the stomach and stop vomiting

Guiding formula: *Li Zhong Tang Jia Wei*

Medicinals: Radix Panacis Ginseng (*Ren Shen*), Rhizoma Atractylodis Macrocephalae (*Bai Zhu*), dry Rhizoma Zingiberis (*Gan Jiang*), Rhizoma Pinelliae Ternatae (*Ban Xia*), Pericarpium Citri Reticulatae (*Chen Pi*), Flos Caryophylli (*Ding Xiang*), Fructus Evodiae Rutecarpae (*Wu Zhu Yu*), mix-fried Radix Glycyrrhizae (*Zhi Gan Cao*)

Formula explanation: Radix Panacis Ginseng, sweet and warm, supplements the center and boosts the qi in order to fortify the normal function of the body. Dry Rhizoma Zingiberis, acrid and hot, warms the center and supports yang, harmonizes the stomach and stops vomiting. Rhizoma Atractylodis Macrocephalae, bitter and warm, dries dampness and fortifies the spleen. Rhizoma Pinelliae Ternatae dries dampness, thus aiding spleen transportation. It also downbears counterflow and stops vomiting. Pericarpium Citri Reticulatae rectifies the qi and fortifies the spleen. Adding Flos Caryophylli warms the middle and scatters cold, downbears counterflow and stops vomiting. Radix Glycyrrhizae rectifies and harmonizes the preceding medicinals.

Selected acupuncture/moxibustion points: *Gong Sun* (Sp 4)⊥, *Guan Yuan* (CV 4)▵, *Zhong Wan* (CV 12)|, & *Shen Que* (Cv 8)▵

Formula rationale: Supplementing *Gong Sun* fortifies the spleen and boosts the stomach, harmonizes the middle and stops vomiting. Needling and then adding moxibustion at *Guan Yuan* warms the yang and boosts the spleen, harmonizes the stomach and downbears counterflow. Moxaing *Shen Que* rouses central yang in order to aid transportation. Even supplementation and drainage of *Zhong Wan* fortifies the spleen, harmonizes the stomach, and stops vomiting.

3. *Tan Yin Nei Ting*
Phlegm Rheum Internally Collected

Clinical manifestations: Vomiting clear water, phlegm, and saliva, epigastric oppression and discomfort, heart palpitations, dizziness, white, slimy tongue fur, and a slippery pulse

Treatment principles: Warm the middle and transform phlegm, harmonize the stomach and stop vomiting

Guiding formula: *Xiao Ban Xia Tang* plus *Ling Gui Zhu Gan Tang*

Medicinals: Rhizoma Pinelliae Ternatae (*Ban Xia*), Sclerotium Poriae Cocos (*Fu Ling*), Cortex Cinnamomi (*Gui Pi*), Rhizoma Atractylodis Macrocephalae (*Bai Zhu*), Pericarpium Citri Reticulatae (*Chen Pi*), uncooked Rhizoma Zingiberis (*Sheng Jiang*)

Formula explanation: Rhizoma Pinelliae Ternatae expels phlegm, harmonizes the stomach, and stops vomiting. Sclerotium Poriae Cocos blandly seeps and fortifies the spleen. Cortex Cinnamomi warms the channels and smoothes the passages of yang. It is combined with uncooked Rhizoma Zingiberis, which warms the middle and stops vomiting. Rhizoma Atractylodis Macrocephalae dries dampness and fortifies the spleen. Pericarpium Citri Reticulatae rectifies the qi and transports the spleen, harmonizes the stomach and transforms phlegm. When these medicinals are used together, they harmonize the middle and transform phlegm, warm the stomach and stop vomiting.

Selected acupuncture/moxibustion points: *Nei Guan* (Per 6)⊥, *Gong Sun* (Sp 4)⊥, *Feng Long* (St 40)⊥, & *Zhong Wan* (CV 12)⊥x

Formula rationale: Both *Nei Guan* and *Gong Sun* are meeting points of the eight vessels which connect with the stomach, heart, and chest. Used together, they fortify the spleen and aid transportation, harmonize the stomach and stop vomiting. Draining *Feng Long* transforms phlegm and aids transportation. Also needling and then adding moxa at *Zhong Wan* warms and transforms phlegm, harmonizes the stomach and stops vomiting.

4. *Wei Yin Bu Zu*
Stomach Yin Insufficiency

Clinical manifestations: Severe vomiting with difficulty eating or even inability to eat or drink, even tiny drops of water not entering, dry mouth and throat, a red tongue with scant fur, and a fine, rapid pulse

Treatment principles: Nourish the stomach and engender fluids, downbear counterflow and stop vomiting

Guiding formula: *Ju Pi Zhu Ru Tang Jia Wei*

Medicinals: Radix Panacis Ginseng (*Ren Shen*), Pericarpium Citri Erythrocarpae (*Ju Pi*), Caulis Bambusae In Taeniis (*Zhu Ru*), Tuber Ophiopogonis Japonicae (*Mai Dong*), Radix Trichosanthis Kirlowii

(*Tian Hua Fen*), Rhizoma Anemarrhenae (*Zhi Mu*), Fructus Zizyphi Jujubae (*Da Zao*), uncooked Rhizoma Zingiberis (*Sheng Jiang*)

Formula explanation: Pericarpium Citri Erythrocarpae rectifies the qi and harmonizes the stomach, downbears counterflow and stops vomiting. Caulis Bambusae In Taeniis clears the stomach and stops vomiting. These two are the ruling medicinals. They are combined with Radix Panacis Ginseng, which greatly supplements source qi, engenders fluids, and stops thirst. Uncooked Rhizoma Zingiberis harmonizes the stomach and stops vomiting. Rhizoma Anemarrhenae and Radix Trichosanthis Kirlowii used together enrich yin and discharge fire, clear heat and engender fluids. Tuber Ophiopogonis Japonicae boosts the stomach and engenders fluids. Radix Glycyrrhizae and Fructus Zizyphi Jujubae boost the qi and harmonize the middle, regulate and harmonize the preceding medicinals.

Selected acupuncture/moxibustion points: *Nei Guan* (Per 6)⊥, *Gong Sun* (Sp 4)⊥, *San Yin Jiao* (Sp 6)⊤, *Fu Liu* (Ki 7)⊤, & *Zu San Li* (St 36)|

Formula rationale: *Nei Guan* above and *Gong Sun* below are combined to harmonize the stomach, downbear counterflow, and stop vomiting. Supplementing *Fu Liu* and *San Yin Jiao* enriches yin, discharges fire, boosts the stomach, and engenders fluids. Even supplementation and drainage of *Zu San Li* fortifies the spleen, boosts the stomach, and balances and rectifies the function of the stomach and intestines.

VI. *Ke Chuan*
Cough & Asthma

Cough and asthma or wheezing are commonly seen respiratory symptoms in AIDS patients. Almost all patients eventually develop various and severe respiratory conditions affecting their bronchi, pleura, pulmonary lobes, and other parts. In full blown AIDS, because of immune system depression and, therefore, lowered resistance to infection, the lungs may easily become infected by *Mycobacterium avium-intracellulara*(MAI), pneumonia, etc. Typically such cases are very serious and are accompanied by asthma and shortness of breath. Breathing is hard pressed and difficult. X-rays usually reveal pathological spots on the lobes which may merge into large areas resulting in dense, soggy, wet, yin shadows.

A. Disease Causes, Disease Mechanisms

According to Chinese medical theory, the causes of this condition are mostly viscera and bowels damage and detriment causing a reduction in the body's ability to combat disease and lung defensive qi not being secured, thus resulting in entry and invasion by external evils. In the early stage, evils attack lung defensive qi causing the lungs to lose their downbearing and dispersion. Lung qi counterflows upward manifesting as cough. In addition, external evils may move internally. Evil heat obstructs the lungs and steaming of fluids becomes phlegm. Phlegm heat depresses and blocks the lungs. Lung qi is inhibited and hence a series of signs appear indicating phlegm heat. Or, spleen qi vacuity and weakness may lead to loss of expulsion and promotion of transportation. Phlegm turbidity is then engenderd internally. Disturbing upwards, this may cause cough. In chronic patients, yin qi may be consumed and damaged. Lung and kidney yin may thus become vacuous. Dispersion and downbearing are then not right and the kidneys fail to grasp the qi. Counterflow of qi thus results in cough and asthma. If a patient's viscera and bowels, and qi and blood decline further and become even more vacuous, the righteous cannot beat the evil, and vacuous yang will be on the verge of desertion. This then is a critical situation.

B. Differentiation & Treatment

1. *Xie Fan Fei Wei*
Evils Attack Lung Defensive Qi

Clinical manifestations: Cough with white or pale yellow phlegm, chest oppression or pain, typically fever, body pain, thirst and sore throat, a red tongue with thin, white or yellow fur, and a floating, rapid pulse

Treatment principles: Course wind and clear heat, diffuse the lungs and transform phlegm

Guiding formula: *Yin Qiao San Jia Jian*

Medicinals: Flos Lonicerae Japonicae (*Yin Hua*), Fructus Forsythiae Suspensae (*Lian Qiao*), Cortex Radicis Mori Albi (*Sang Bai Pi*), Pericarpium Trichosanthis Kirlowii (*Gua Lou Pi*), Radix Scutellariae Baicalensis (*Huang Qin*), Herba Menthae Haplocalycis (*Bo He*), Semen Pruni Armeniacae (*Xing Ren*), Rhizoma Belamcandae (*She Gan*), Radix Glycyrrhizae (*Gan Cao*)

Formula explanation: Flos Lonicerae Japonicae and Fructus Forsythiae Suspensae clear heat and resolve toxins, gently diffuse the lungs and out-thrust the exterior. Radix Platycodi Grandiflori (*Jie Geng*) and Herba Menthae Haplocalycis gently clear and diffuse the lungs and expel phlegm. Cortex Radicis Mori Albi and Pericarpium Trichosanthis Kirlowii clear the lungs, transform phlegm, and level asthma. Rhizoma Belamcandae clears heat, resolves toxins, and disinhibits the throat. Adding Semen Pruni Armeniacae stops coughing and levels asthma. Radix Scutellariae Baicalensis clears lung heat. And Radix Glycyrrhizae regulates and harmonizes the preceding medicinals.

Selected acupuncture/moxibustion points: *Lie Que* (Lu 7)⊥, *Da Zhui* (GV 14)⊥, *Fei Shu* (Bl 13)|, *He Gu* (LI 4)⊥, & *Feng Chi* (GB 20)|

Formula rationale: Draining *Lie Que* diffuses the lungs and stops coughing. *Da Zhui* is the meeting point of the yang channels and the *du mai*. It aids the yang and resolves toxins. Even supplementation and drainage of *Feng Chi* courses wind and scatters heat in order to eliminate wind evils. *Fei Shu* clears the lungs and stops coughing. Draining *He Gu* courses wind and resolves the exterior, clears heat and diffuses the lungs.

2. *Tan Re Yong Fei*
Phlegm Heat Obstructs the Lungs

Clinical manifestations: High fever, coughing and spitting up yellow phlegm, thick and strong tasting, chest oppression, labored breathing, short, yellow urine, a red tongue with yellow fur, and a surging, big or slippery, rapid pulse

Treatment principles: Clear heat and resolve toxins, diffuse the lungs and transform phlegm

Guiding formula: *Qing Jin Hua Tan Tang Jia Jian*

Medicinals: Rhizoma Coptidis Chinensis (*Huang Lian*), Radix Scutellariae Baicalensis (*Huang Qin*), Cortex Radicis Lycii Chinensis (*Di Gu Pi*), Cortex Radicis Mori Albi (*Sang Bai Pi*), Fructus Gardeniae Jasminoidis (*Shan Zhi*), Semen Pruni Armeniacae (*Xing Ren*), Radix Glycyrrhizae (*Sheng Gan Cao*), Bulbus Fritillariae Thunbergii (*Bei Mu*), Fructus Trichosanthis Kirlowii (*Gua Lou*), Tuber Ophiopogonis Japonicae (*Mai Dong*)

Formula explanation: In this formula, Cortex Radicis Mori Albi drains the lungs and levels asthma. Rhizoma Coptidis Chinensis and Radix Scutellariae Baicalensis are chosen to clear heat and resolve toxins, clear and drain lung heat. Fructus Gardeniae Jasminoidis clears heat and disinhibits dampness, cools the blood and resolves toxins. Tuber Ophiopogonis Japonicae enriches yin, moistens the lungs, and engenders fluids. Bitter Semen Pruni Armeniacae downbears and stops cough and levels asthma. Cortex Radicis Lycii Chinensis clears and discharges lung heat. This is aided by Bulbus Fritillariae Thunbergii and Fructus Trichosanthis Kirlowii which clear the lungs and transform phlegm. Radix Glycyrrhizae clears heat and resolves toxins, regulates and harmonizes the preceding medicinals.

Selected acupuncture/moxibustion points: *Lie Que* (Lu 7)⊥, *Feng Long* (St 40)⊥, *Nei Ting* (St 44)⊥, *Chi Ze* (Lu 5)↓, & *Qu Chi* (LI 11)⊥

Formula rationale: Draining *Lie Que* clears the lungs and transforms phlegm, diffuses the lungs and stops cough. Bleeding *Chi Ze* discharges lung heat. *Feng Long* clears and transforms phlegm heat. *Nei Ting* is the spring point of the foot *yang ming*. It clears and discharges internal heat. *Qu Chi* clears heat and resolves toxins.

3. *Fei Pi Qi Xu*
Lung/Spleen Qi Vacuity

Clinical manifestations: Coughing without force, the sound of phlegm in the throat, wheezing not obvious, a lustreless facial complexion, low fever with sweating, mind not buoyed up, or diarrhea or very loose stools, a pale tongue with a white, slimy fur, and a fine, forceless pulse

Treatment principles: Fortify the spleen and supplement the lungs, boost the qi and stop coughing

Guiding formula: *Liu Jun Zi Tang* plus *Bu Fei Tang Jia Jian*

Medicinals: Radix Codonopsis Pilosulae (*Dang Shen*), Rhizoma Atractylodis Macrocephalae (*Bai Zhu*), Sclerotium Poriae Cocos (*Fu Ling*), Rhizoma Pinelliae Ternatae (*Ban Xia*), Pericarpium Citri Reticulatae (*Chen Pi*), Radix Astragali Membranacei (*Huang Qi*), prepared Radix Rehmanniae (*Shu Di*), Fructus Schizandrae Chinensis (*Wu Wei Zi*), Cortex Radicis Mori Albi (*Sang Bai Pi*), Radix Asteris Tatarici (*Zi Wan*)

Formula explanation: In this formula, Rhizoma Pinelliae Ternatae and Sclerotium Poriae dry dampness and transform phlegm, fortify the spleen and aid transportation. Pericarpium Citri Reticulatae regulates the qi and transforms phlegm. Radix Astragali Membranacei supplements lung and spleen qi. Prepared Radix Rehmanniae nourishes the blood and enriches yin in order to supplement vacuity. Fructus Schizandrae Chinensis takes in and restrains lung qi. Radix Asteris Tatarici and Cortex Radicis Mori Albi transform phlegm and stop coughing. Radix Glycyrrhizae harmonizes the middle and regulates and harmonizes the preceding medicinals. Used together, the above medicinals fortify the spleen and supplement the lungs, transform phlegm and stop coughing.

Selected acupuncture/moxibustion points: *Pi Shu* (Bl 20)т, *Fei Shu* (Bl 13)т, *Zu San Li* (St 36)т, *Tai Yuan* (Lu 9)т, & *Tai Bai* (Sp 3)т

Formula rationale: *Pi Shu* and *Fei Shu* are back *shu* points. They are chosen to supplement the spleen and boost the lungs, banking earth to engender metal. *Zu San Li* fortifies the spleen and aids transportation, supplements and boosts the postnatal. *Tai Yuan* is the source point of the lung channel. It supplements the lungs and boosts the qi, expels phlegm and levels asthma. *Tai Bai* is the source point of the spleen. Its functions are to fortify the spleen and boost the stomach, boost the qi and conserve the blood. Used together, these points can supplement the spleen and boost the lungs, level asthma and stop coughing.

4. *Fei Shen Yin Xu*
Lung/Kidney Yin Vacuity

Clinical manifestations: Cough with scant phlegm or cough with no phlegm, qi counterflow, labored breathing, tidal fever and night sweats, vacuity vexation and insomnia, bodily emaciation, dry mouth and throat, a red tongue with scant fur, and a fine, rapid pulse

Treatment principles: Nourish yin and clear heat, moisten the lungs and stop coughing

Guiding formula: *Sha Shen Mai Dong Tang Jia Jian*

Medicinals: Radix Glehniae Littoralis (*Sha Shen*), Tuber Ophiopogonis Japonicae (*Mai Dong*), Rhizoma Polygonati Odorati (*Yu Zhu*), Folium Mori Albi Albi (*Sang Ye*), Bulbus Fritillariae (*Bei Mu*), Radix Trichosanthis Kirlowii (*Tian Hua Fen*), prepared Radix Rehmanniae (*Shu Di*), Cortex Radicis Moutan (*Dan Pi*), Rhizoma Alismatis (*Ze Xie*), Radix Glycyrrhizae (*Gan Cao*)

Formula explanation: Using Radix Glehniae Littoralis, Tuber Ophiopogonis Japonicae, Rhizoma Polygonati Odorati, and Radix Trichosanthis Kirlowii nourishes yin and moistens the lungs, engenders fluids and stops thirst. Prepared Radix Rehmanniae enriches and supplements kidney yin. Bulbus Fritillariae Thunbergii clears the lungs, transforms phlegm, and stops coughing. Cortex Radicis Moutan and Rhizoma Alismatis clear and discharge lung and kidney fire. Radix Glycyrrhizae regulates and harmonizes the preceding medicinals. Used together, these medicinals are able to enrich and supplement lung and kidney yin, clear heat, and stop coughing.

Selected acupuncture/moxibustion points: *Tai Xi* (Ki 3)⊤, *Fei Shu* (Bl 13)⊤, *Shen Shu* (Bl 23)⊤, *Zu San Li* (St 36)⊤, & *Fu Liu* (Ki 7)⊤

Formula rationale: Supplementing *Tai Xi* and *Fu Liu* enriches and supplements lung and kidney yin, enriches yin and clears heat. *Fei Shu* and *Shen Shu* are chosen to supplement and boost the lungs and kidneys, stop coughing and level asthma. Supplementing *Zu San Li* fortifies the spleen and boosts the qi, transforms phlegm and aids transportation.

5. *Yang Xu Yu Tuo*
Yang Vacuity on the Verge of Desertion

Clinical manifestations: Facial complexion suddenly somber white, cold sweat dribbling and dripping, breathing short and labored, cold inversion of the four limbs, a pale tongue, and a faint pulse on the verge of severance

Treatment principles: Boost the qi, return yang, and secure desertion

Guiding formula: *Shen Fu Tang Jia Wei*

Medicinals: Radix Panacis Ginseng (*Ren Shen*), Radix Lateralis Praeparatus Aconiti Carmicheali (*Fu Zi*), Os Draconis (*Long Gu*), Concha Ostreae (*Mu Li*), mix-fried Radix Glycyrrhizae (*Zhi Gan Cao*)

Formula explanation: Radix Panacis Ginseng greatly supplements the source qi. Radix Lateralis Praeparatus Aconiti Carmichaeli, extremely acrid, extremely warm, warms and invigorates yang qi. These two medicinals used together return yang and secure desertion. Adding Os Draconis and Concha Ostreae grasps, restrains, secures, and astringes as well as has the ability to quiet the spirit. Radix Praeparatus Glycyrrhizae fortifies the spleen and harmonizes the middle, regulates and harmonizes the preceding medicinals.

Selected acupuncture/moxibustion points: *Guan Yuan* (CV 4)▲, *Qi Hai* (CV 6)▲, *Shen Men* (Ht 7)⊤, & *Bai Hui* (GV 20)⊤x

Formula rationale: Moxaing *Guan Yuan* and *Qi Hai* warms and supplements the lower source, boosts the qi, returns yang, and secures desertion. Supplementing *Shen Men* tranquilizes the heart and quiets the spirit, boosts the qi and revives the pulse. Supplementing *Ba Hui* by needling and then applying moxibustion boosts the qi and upbears yang, returns yang and secures desertion.

VII. *Zi Han Dao Han*
Spontaneous Perspiration & Night Sweats

Night sweats and spontaneous perspiration are both pathoconditions associated with the AIDS prodromal stage. Sometimes there is night sweating commonly accompanied by fever, and sometimes spontaneous perspiration appears. Their etiology is not clear.

A. Disease Causes, Disease Mechanisms

As early as the *Nei Jing*, the physiology and pathophysiology of sweating were well understood. Sweat is the fluid of the heart. The kidneys rule the five fluids. Owing to internal invasion of pestilential toxic evils, the viscera and bowels are deficient and vacuous. This causes yin and yang to lose their regulation. There is vacuity and weakness of the qi and blood. The defensive qi is not secured and this leads to sweat and fluids being discharged externally. If lung qi is vacuous and weak, the *wei wai* or defensive exterior is unsecured. This also may cause spontaneous perspiration. If evil toxins injure yin and kidney yin is deficient and vacuous, vacuous fire will be engenderd internally. Yin fluids will be disturbed and will not be able to be treasured or stored internally. Rather they will be discharged outwardly as night sweats. In prolonged cases, vacuity of both qi and yin may cause the alternating appearance of night sweats and spontaneous perspiration.

B. Differentiation & Treatment

1. *Wei Biao Bu Gu*
Defensive Exterior Not Secured

Clinical manifestations: Sweating with fear of wind or drafts, increased sweating with exertion, lassitude of the spirit, lack of strength, a lustreless facial complexion, mouth bland and tasteless, no thirst, possible loose stools or diarrhea, a pale tongue with thin, light fur, and a fine, weak pulse

Treatment principles: Boost the qi, secure the exterior, and stop sweating

Guiding formula: *Yu Ping Feng San Jia Wei*

Medicinals: Radix Astragali Membranacei (*Huang Qi*), Rhizoma Atractylodis Macrocephalae (*Bai Zhu*), Radix Ledebouriellae Sesloidis (*Fang Feng*), Fructus Levis Tritici Aestivi (*Fu Xiao Mai*), Concha Ostreae (*Mu Li*), Radix Codonopsis Pilosulae (*Dang Shen*)

Formula explanation: In this formula, Radix Astragali Membranacei boosts the qi, secures the exterior, and stops sweating. Therefore it is used as the ruling medicinal in this formula. Rhizoma Atractylodis Macrocephalae fortifies the spleen and eliminates dampness. It aids Radix Astragali Membranacei in boosting the qi and securing the exterior. Adding a little Radix Ledebouriellae Sesloidis expels the exterior and carefully scatters evils. It aids Radix Astragali Membranacei in securing the exterior and expels winds. Adding Concha Ostreae and Fructus Levis Tritici Aestivi holds, restrains, secures, and astringes and stops sweating. Combining these ingredients with Radix Codonopsis Pilosulae strengthens this formula's ability to boost the qi and fortify the spleen.

Selected acupuncture/moxibustion points: *He Gu* (LI 4)т, *Qi Hai* (CV 6)ᴀ, *Zu San Li* (St 36)т, *San Yin Jiao* (Sp 6)т, & *Fu Liu* (Ki 7)т

Formula ratonale: Supplementing *He Gu* boosts the qi and secures the exterior, upbear and lifts yang qi. *He Gu* and *Fu Liu* used together are able to secure the exterior and stop sweating. Supplementing *San Yin Jiao* enriches yin and engenders blood in order to aid the source of sweat. *Zu San Li* boosts the qi and fortifies the spleen, banks earth to engender metal. Needling *Qi Hai* followed by moxa strongly supplements the source qi, warms the yang, and boosts the qi. Used together, these points boost the qi, secure the exterior, and stop sweating.

2. *Yin Xu Huo Wang*
Yin Vacuity, Fire Effulgence

Clinical manifestations: Tidal fever and night sweats, both cheeks red, vexatious heat in the five hearts, dizziness, tinnitus, loss of sleep, excessive dreaming, a red tongue with scant fur, a fine, rapid pulse

Treatment principles: Enrich yin and downbear fire

Guiding formula: *Dang Gui Liu Huang Tang*

Medicinals: Radix Angelicae Sinensis (*Dang Gui*), uncooked Radix Rehmanniae (*Sheng Di*), prepared Radix Rehmanniae (*Shu Di*), Rhizoma Coptidis Chinensis (*Huang Lian*), Radix Scutellariae Baicalensis (*Huang Qin*), Cortex Phellodendri (*Huang Bai*), Concha Ostreae (*Mu Li*), Fructus Levis Tritici Aestivi (*Fu Xiao Mai*), Radix Astragali Membranacei (*Huang Qi*)

Formula explanation: The medicinals Radix Angelicae Sinensis and prepared Radix Rehmanniae are chosen to nourish yin and supplement the blood. Uncooked Radix Rehmanniae clears heat and cools the blood, nourishes yin and engenders fluids. The combination of Rhizoma Coptidis Chinensis, Radix Scutellariae Baicalensis, and Cortex Phellodendri clears heat, discharges fire, and relieves vexation. Radix Astragali Membranacei boosts the qi and secures the exterior. Concha Ostreae and Fructus Levis Tritici Aestivi hold, restrain, secure, and astringe and stop sweating. Used together, these medicinals enrich yin and discharge heat, secure the exterior and stop sweating.

Selected acupuncture/moxibustion points: *Tai Xi* (Ki 3)⊤, *Yin Xi* (Ht 6)⊥, *Hou Xi* (SI 3)⊥, *Fu Liu* (Ki 7)⊤, & *Tai Chong* (Liv 3)⊥

Formula rationale: The source point of the kidney channel is chosen to enrich and supplement kidney yin. *Yin Xi*, the river point of the hand *shao yin* channel, is chosen to clear and discharge heart fire. When combined with *Hou Xi* and drained, they effectively treat night sweats. Supplementing *Fu Liu* enriches and supplements kidney water. Draining *Tai Chong* levels the liver and discharges fire. Used together, these points enrich yin and downbear fire.

3. *Qi Yin Liang Xu*
Qi & Yin Dual Vacuity

Clinical manifestations: Tidal fever and night sweats commonly accompanied by spontaneous perspiration, copious discharge of sweat, shortness of breath, lack of strength, heart vexation with little sleep, hand, foot, and heart heat, dry mouth, a pale tongue with scant fur, and a fine, weak pulse

Treatment principles: Boost the qi and nourish yin

Guiding formula: *Sheng Mai San Jia Wei*

Medicinals: Radix Panacis Ginseng (*Ren Shen*), Tuber Ophiopogonis Japonicae (*Mai Dong*), Fructus Schizandrae Chinensis (*Wu Wei Zi*),

Carapax Amydae Sinensis (*Bei Jia*), Cortex Radicis Lycii Chinensis (*Di Gu Pi*), Rhizoma Anemarrhenae (*Zhi Mu*), Fructus Levis Tritici Aestivi (*Fu Xiao Mai*), prepared Radix Rehmanniae (*Shu Di*), Radix Praeparatus Glycyrrhizae (*Zhi Gan Cao*)

Formula explanation: In this formula, Radix Panacis Ginseng greatly supplements source qi, boosts the qi, and engenders fluids. It is combined with Tuber Ophiopogonis Japonicae which nourishes yin, clears heat, and engenders fluids. Fructus Schizandrae Chinensis restrains the lungs, stops sweating, and engenders fluids. Fructus Levis Tritici Aestivi boosts the qi and stops sweating. Prepared Radix Rehmanniae enriches yin and supplements the kidneys. Carapax Amydae Sinensis and Rhizoma Anemarrhenae enrich yin and clear heat. Cortex Radicis Lycii Chinensis effectively clears vacuous heat. And Radix Praeparatus Glycyrrhizae regulates and harmonizes the preceding medicinals.

Selected acupuncture/moxibustion points: *Fu Liu* (Ki 7)⊤, *Yin Xi* (Ht 6)⊥, *He Gu* (LI 4)⊤, *Qi Hai* (CV 6)⊤, & *Tai Xi* (Ki 3)⊤

Formula rationale: *Fu Liu* is chosen to enrich and boost kidney water. Draining *Yin Xi* clears heart fire. Used together, they enrich kidney yin and stop night sweats. Supplementing *He Gu* boosts the qi and secures the exterior. *Qi Hai* cultivates and supplements source qi. Used together, these points secure the exterior and stop sweating. *Tai Xi* enriches yin and supplements the kidneys.

VIII. *Shi Mian*
Loss of Sleep or Insomnia

Insomnia is one of the mostly commonly seen symptoms in the course of AIDS. Owing to patients' psychological fear of this disease, their minds are not steady or stable and lack calm. Typically, they display worry and anxiety, vexation and agitittation, etc. This results in excitation of the brain cortex. If this state persists for some time, there will be neurasthenia, *i.e.*, long-standing insomnia. If insomnia is constant, it will affect the patient's mind and nervous system negatively. This will inhibit treatment and even cause the patient's condition to deengender.

A. Disease Causes, Disease Mechanisms

Insomnia (*shi mian*, literally loss of sleep) is also called *bu mei* or "not sleeping". There are many reasons for its onset. However, almost all AIDS' insomnia is caused by none other than heart, spleen, and kidney deficiency and vacuity or loss of emotional equilibrium. If there is dual heart/spleen vacuity, the origin of creation and transformation will be insufficient. Yin blood is consumed and is unable to offer upwards to the heart. Heart spirit loses nourishment resulting in the heart spirit not being tranquil and, thus, insomnia. If heart yin is deficient and vacuous, heart yang will tends towards effulgence. Yin cannot control yang. Heart spirit is not quiet and cannot enter sleep. If kidney yin is deficient and vacuous, kidney water will not be able to restrain heart fire flaring above. Heart fire will separate from its source and the mind will not be tranquil. Hence insomnia. Because of fear of this disease, the liver may be injured by depression. If the liver loses its ability to promote coursing and discharge, depression may transform into fire which harasses and injures the spirit brilliance. When the spirit is not quiet or tranquil, sleep also is not quiet. Further, if the patient dreads this disease and lives in fear every day, there will be heart vacuity and gallbladder timidity which also may contribute to the causation of insomnia.

B. Differentiation & Treatment

1. *Xin Pi Liang Xu*
Heart/Spleen Dual Vacuity

Clinical manifestations: Loss of sleep, profuse dreaming, heart palpitations, impaired memory, lassitude of the spirit, lack of strength, diminshed lustre of the facial complexion, poor appetite, epigastric oppression, loose stools, a pale tongue with a thin, white fur, and a fine, weak pulse

Treatment principles: Fortify the spleen and boost the qi, supplement the heart and nourish blood

Guiding formula: *Gui Pi Tang Jia Wei*

Medicinals: Radix Panacis Ginseng (*Ren Shen*), Rhizoma Atractylodis Macrocephalae (*Bai Zhu*), Radix Astragali Membranacei (*Huang Qi*), Radix Polygalae Tenuifoliae (*Yuan Zhi*), Semen Zizyphi Spinosae (*Suan Zao Ren*), Sclerotium Parardicis Poriae Cocos (*Fu Shen*), Arillus Euphoriae Longanae (*Long Yan Rou*), Radix Angelicae Sinensis (*Dang Gui*), Radix Saussureae Seu Valadimiriae (*Mu Xiang*), Radix Praeparatus Glycyrrhizae (*Zhi Gan Cao*)

Formula explanation: In this formula, *Si Jun Tang* supplements the qi and fortifies the spleen. Radix Astragali Membranacei boosts the qi. Radix Angelicae Sinensis supplements and activates the blood. Radix Polygalae Tenuifoliae, Semen Zizyphi Spinosae, and Arillus Euphoriae Longanae nourish the heart and quiet the spirit. Radix Auklandiae regulates the qi, fortifies the spleen, and aids transportation so that supplementation does not cause stagnation. Uncooked Rhizoma Zingiberis (*Sheng Jiang*) and Fructus Zizyphi Jujubae (*Da Zao*) regulate and harmonize the constructive and defensive. Together, these medicinals supplement the qi and engender blood as well as quiet the heart spirit. This automatically stops loss of sleep.

Selected acupuncture/moxibustion points: *Shen Men* (Ht 7)т, *San Yin Jiao* (Sp 6)т, *Xin Shu* (Bl 15)т, & *Zu San Li* (St 36)т

Formula rationale: *Shen Men* is the source point of the heart channel. Supplementing it nourishes the heart and quiets the spirit. Supplementing *San Yin Jiao* enriches yin and engenders blood. Supplementing *Xin Shu* supplements the blood and tranquilizes the heart. *Zu San Li* fortifies the spleen in order to boost the qi and engender blood. Together these points have the ability to supplement and boost the spleen and heart as well as nourish the heart and quiet the spirit.

2. *Xin Yin Kui Xu*
Heart Yin Deficiency & Vacuity

Clinical manifestations: Sleep at night not quiet, profuse dreaming, easily awakened, dizziness, tinnitus, heart palpitations, impaired memory, dry mouth and throat, heat in the hands, feet, and heart, tidal fever, night sweats, a red tongue with scant fur, and a fine, rapid pulse

Treatment principles: Enrich yin and clear heat, nourish the heart and quiet the spirit

Guiding formula: *Tian Wang Bu Xin Dan Jia Wei*

Medicinals: Uncooked Radix Rehmanniae (*Sheng Di*), Radix Panacis Ginseng (*Ren Shen*), Radix Scrophulariae Ningpoensis (*Yuan Shen*), Radix Salviae Miltiorrhizae (*Dan Shen*), Tuber Ophiopogonis Japonicae (*Mai Dong*), Tuber Asparagi Cochinensis (*Tian Dong*), Sclerotium Poriae Cocos (*Fu Ling*), Fructus Schizandrae Chinensis (*Wu Wei Zi*), Radix Polygalae Tenuifoliae (*Yuan Zhi*), Semen Biotae Orientalis (*Bai Zi Ren*), Semen Zizyphi Spinosae (*Suan Zao Ren*), Cinnabar (*Zhu Sha*)

Formula explanation: In this formula, uncooked Radix Rehmanniae, Radix Scrophulariae Nongpoensis, Tuber Asparagi Cochinensis, and Tuber Ophiopogonis Japonicae, all sweet, cold, enriching, and moistening, supplement yin and engender fluids. Radix Salviae Miltiorrhizae and Radix Angelicae Sinensis supplement and quicken the blood in order to nourish the heart. Radix Codonopsis Pilosulae (*Dang Shen*) and Sclerotium Poriae Cocos boost the qi and fortify the spleen. Semen Biotae Orientalis, Radix Polygalae Tenuifoliae, and Semen Zizyphi Spinosae nourish the heart and quiet the spirit. Cinnabaris clears heat, heavily settles the heart, and quiets the spirit. Fructus Schizandrae Chinensis enriches yin and engenders fluids, tranquilizes the heart and quiets the spirit.

Selected acupuncture/moxibustion points: *Shen Men* (Ht 7)⊤, *Yin Xi* (Ht 6)⊥, *Xue Hai* (Sp 10)⊤, & *Tai Xi* (Ki 3)⊤

Formula rationale: Supplementing *Shen Men* nourishes heart yin and tranquilizes the heart spirit. Draining *Yin Xi* clears the heart and downbears fire. Supplementing *Xue Hai* supplements the blood and nourishes the heart. Also it can supplement the blood, enrich yin, and quicken the blood. Supplementing *Tai Xi* enriches and supplements kidney yin and, therefore, nourishes heart yin.

3. *Yin Xu Huo Wang*
Yin Vacuity, Fire Effulgence

Clinical manifestations: Heart vexation, loss of sleep, sometimes not sleeping all night, dizziness, tinnitus, impaired memory, profuse dreaming, low back and knee soreness and weakness, seminal emission, tidal fever, night sweats, vexatious heat in the five hearts, a red tongue with scant fur, and a fine, rapid pulse

Treatment principles: Enrich the kidneys and downbear fire, nourish the heart and quiet the spirit

Guiding formula: *Huang Lian E Jiao Tang Jia Wei*

Medicinals: Rhizoma Coptidis Chinensis (*Huang Lian*), Gelatinum Corii Asini (*E Jiao*), Radix Scutellariae Baicalensis (*Huang Qin*), Radix Albus Paeoniae Lactiflorae (*Bai Shao*), prepared Radix Rehmanniae (*Shu Di*), Semen Biotae Orientalis (*Bai Zi Ren*), Semen Zizyphi Spinosae (*Suan Zao Ren*)

Formula explanation: Rhizoma Coptidis Chinensis clears heat and resolves toxins, thus relieving vexation. Gelatinum Corii Asini enriches yin and nourishes blood. Radix Scutellariae Baicalensis aids Rhizoma Coptidis Chinensis in clearing and eliminating heat evils. Radix Albus Paeoniae Lactiflorae nourishes the blood and astringes yin. Semen Zizyphi Spinosae and Semen Biotae Orientalis nourish the heart and quiet the spirit. Prepared Radix Rehmanniae enriches and supplements kidney yin. Used together, these medicinals have the ability to enrich the kidneys and downbear fire, nourish the heart and quiet the spirit.

Selected acupuncture/moxibustion points: *Shen Men* (Ht 7)⊥, *Fu Liu* (Ki 7)⊤, *Tai Xi* (Ki 3)⊤, & *San Yin Jiao* (Sp 6)⊤

Formula ratonale: Needling and draining *Shen Men* clears the heart and discharges fire, tranquilizes the heart and quiets the spirit. Supplementing *Fu Liu* enriches yin water. *Tai Xi* connects freely the heart and kidneys, guiding fire to gather at its source. And *San Yin Jiao* enriches the blood and engenders fluids. Used together, these points enrich yin, downbear fire, and quiet the heart spirit.

4. *Gan Yu Hua Huo*
Liver Depression Transforms into Fire

Clinical manifestations: Sleep not quiet, profuse dreaming, easily awakened, heart vexation not quiet, no thought of food or drink, chest oppression, fullness, and distention, sighing, a bitter taste in the mouth, short, yellowish urine, a red tongue with yellow fur, and a wiry, rapid pulse

Treatment principles: Course the liver and discharge fire, clear heat and quiet the mind

Guiding formula: *Long Dan Xie Gan Tang Jia Wei*

Medicinals: Radix Gentianae Scabrae (*Long Dan Cao*), Fructus Gardeniae Jasminoidis (*Zhi Zi*), Radix Scutellariae Baicalensis (*Huang Qin*), Rhizoma Alismatis (*Ze Xie*), Caulis Akebiae (*Mu Tong*), Semen Plantaginis (*Che Qian Zi*), Radix Bupleuri (*Chai Hu*), Radix Angelicae Sinensis (*Dang Gui*), uncooked Radix Rehmanniae (*Sheng Di*), Os Draconis (*Long Gu*), Concha Margaritiferae (*Zhen Zhu Mu*), Radix Glycyrrhizae (*Gan Cao*)

Formula explanation: In this formula, Radix Gentianae Scabrae discharges liver/gallbladder fire. Fructus Gardeniae Jasminoidis, cold and bitter, discharges fire and assists Radix Gentianae Scabrae in discharging liver/gallbladder full heat. Rhizoma Alismatis and Caulis Akebiae clear and disinhibit damp heat, leading out fire via urination.

Radix Angelicae Sinensis and uncooked Radix Rehmanniae nourish the blood and harmonize the liver. Radix Bupleuri courses liver/gallbladder qi. Radix Glycyrrhizae harmonizes the middle. Adding Os Draconis and Concha Margaritiferae heavily settles and quiets the spirit. Used together, these medicinals eliminate liver fire. Thus the heart spirit automatically becomes quiet.

Selected acupuncture/moxibustion points: *Shen Men* (Ht 7)⊥, *Tai Chong* (Liv 3)⊥, *Nei Guan* (Per 6)⊥, & *Tai Xi* (Ki 3)⊤

Formula rationale: Needling and draining *Shen Men* clears the heart and quiets the spirit. *Tai Chong* courses the liver and discharges fire. Draining *Nei Guan* broadens the chest and regulates the qi, clears the heart and quiets the spirit. Supplementing *Tai Xi* enriches kidney yin and levels heart fire.

5. *Xin Dan Qi Xu*
Heart/Gallbladder Qi Vacuity

Clinical manifestations: No sleep, profuse dreaming, easily awakened in a start, dizziness, blurred vision, shortness of breath, lack of strength, long, clear urine, a pale, fat tongue, and a fine, weak pulse

Treatment principles: Boost the qi, quiet the spirit, and stabilize the emotions

Guiding formula: *An Shen Ding Zhi Wan Jia Jian*

Medicinals: Radix Panacis Ginseng (*Ren Shen*), Semen Zizyphi Spinosae (*Suan Zao Ren*), Radix Albus Paeoniae Lactiflorae (*Bai Shao*), Caulis Bambusae In Taeniis (*Zhu Ru*), Sclerotium Poriae Cocos (*Fu Ling*), Radix Polygalae Tenuifoliae (*Yuan Zhi*), Rhizoma Acori Graminei (*Shi Chang Pu*), Dens Draconis (*Long Yan*), Sclerotium Pararadicis Poriae Cocos (*Fu Shen*)

Formula explanation: In this formula, Radix Panacis Ginseng boosts the qi and nourishes the heart. Dens Draconis heavily settles, stills, and quiets the spirit. Sclerotium Poriae Cocos boosts the qi and fortifies the spleen. Sclerotium Pararadicis Poriae Cocos and Rhizoma Acori Graminei supplement the qi, boost the gallbladder, and quiet the spirit. Radix Polygalae Tenuifoliae and Semen Zizyphi Spinosae tranquilize the heart and quiet the spirit. Radix Albus Paeoniae Lactiflorae, sour and sweet, is chosen to transform yin and thus nourish heart blood. Adding a little Caulis Bambusae In Taeniis clears the heart and eliminates vexation.

Selected acupuncture/moxibustion points: *Xin Shu* (Bl 15)⊤, *Shen Men* (Ht 7)⊥, *Da Ling* (Per 7)⊥, & *Zu San Li* (St 36)⊤

Formula rationale: *Xin Shu* is chosen to supplement heart blood. Draining *Shen Men* and *Da Ling* heavily settles the heart, quiets the spirit and emotions. *Zu San Li* boosts the qi, engenders blood, and nourishes the heart. Used together, these points boost the qi, nourish the heart, and quiet the spirit. Thus this condition is automatically relieved.

IX. *Luo Li*
Scrofula, *i.e.*, Lymphadenopathy

During the ARC stage, many patients have lymph node swelling of the entire body without any obvious cause. In most cases, lymph node enlargement is long-standing with some cases continuing for several years. On examination, one may find swollen lymph nodes from 0.5-5.0 cm in size in the neck, armpits, and/or occipital regions, some of which may be tender. In full blown AIDS, due to extremely low immunity, patients often have swollen lymph nodes due to malignant lymphoma.

A. Disease Causes, Disease Mechanisms

TCM classifies this disease as *luo li* or "scrofula". Those nodulations affecting the neck and hypochondrium are called sabre and string of beads respectively. The causes are none other than viscera and bowel deficiency and vacuity, loss of normalcy in coursing, discharging, transporting, and transforming functions, infection by external invading toxic evils, or phlegm dampness stopping and accumulating and mutually bound up with evil toxins which then turn into scrofula. Its root cause is viscera and bowel deficiency and vacuity with phlegm dampness as its outward sign. If there is liver depression and qi stagnation, the spleen may lose its promotion of transportation. Phlegm dampness congeals and obstructs the channels and network vessels. Or, if kidney yin is deficient and vacuous, liver fire may become excessive and arrogant. Fire may burn the fluids and humors into phlegm and phlegm turbidity then congeals and stagnates. This can give rise to scrofula. In chronic AIDS cases, the qi and blood are extremely deficient and vacuous. If stasis accumulates and phlegm congeals, this may result in scrofula and malignant kernels or tumors.

B. Differentiation & Treatment

1. *Qi Zhi Tan Ning*
Qi Stagnation, Phlegm Congelation

Clinical manifestations: Nodulation all over the body accompanied by emotional depression, chest and flank distention and pain, epigastric oppression, poor appetite, a pale tongue with thin fur, and a wiry pulse

Treatment principles: Course the liver and resolve depression, transform phlegm and scatter nodulation

Guiding formula: *Nei Xiao Luo Li Wan Jia Jian*

Medicinals: Spica Prunellae Vulgaris (*Xia Gu Cao*), Radix Bupleuri (*Chai Hu*), Radix Scrophulariae Ningpoensis (*Yuan Shen*), Herba

Sargassii (*Hai Zao*), Bulbus Fritillariae Thunbergii (*Bei Mu*), Radix Trichosanthis Kirlowii (*Hua Fen*), Herba Menthae Haplocalycis (*Bo He*), uncooked Radix Rehmanniae (*Sheng Di*), Radix Angelicae Sinensis (*Dang Gui*), Radix Platycodi Grandiflori (*Jie Geng*), Radix Glycyrrhizae (*Gan Cao*)

Formula explanation: In this formula, Spica Prunellae Vulgaris resolves toxins and transforms phlegm. Radix Bupleuri courses the liver and resolves depression. Radix Scrophulariae Ningpoensis enriches yin, clears heat, and resolves toxins. Herba Sargassii and Bulbus Fritillariae Thunbergii transform phlegm, soften the hard, and scatter nodulation. Radix Trichosanthis Kirlowii and Radix Platycodi Grandiflori resolve toxins, transform phlegm, and disperse swelling. Uncooked Radix Rehmanniae and Radix Angelicae Sinensis enrich yin and nourish the blood. Herba Menthae Haplocalycis, light, clear, diffusing, and scattering, courses the liver and resolves depression. Radix Glycyrrhizae regulates and harmonizes the preceding medicinals.

Selected acupuncture/moxibustion points: *Zhang Men* (Liv 13)⊥, *Tian Jing* (TH 10)⊥, *Zu Lin Qi* (GB 41)⊥, & *Feng Long* (St 40)⊥

Formula rationale: *Zhang Men* is the front *mu* point of the spleen. Draining it discharges the gallbladder, courses the liver, fortifies the spleen, and transforms dampness in order to eliminate phlegm. *Tian Jing* is an empirical point for the treatment of scrofula. Also, draining it is able to clear and disinhibit the three burners, course and disinhibit the qi mechanism. *Zu Lin Qi* is the stream point of the gallbladder channel. It courses and discharges the liver/gallbladder and is good for treating scrofula. Draining *Feng Long* transforms phlegm and scatters nodulation.

2. *Yin Xu Nei Re*
Yin Vacuity, Internal Heat

Clinical manifestations: Scrofula all over accompanied by tidal fever and night sweats, vacuous vexation, not sleeping, dizziness, lassitude of the spirit, dry mouth, vexatious heat in the five hearts, a red tongue with scant fur, and a fine, rapid pulse

Treatment principles: Enrich yin and downbear fire, soften the hard and scatter nodulation

Guiding formula: *Da Bu Yin Wan Jia Jian*

Medicinals: Rhizoma Anemarrhenae (*Zhi Mu*), prepared Radix Rehmanniae (*Shu Di*), Cortex Phellodendri (*Huang Bai*), Plastrum Testudinis (*Gui Ban*), Radix Scrophulariae Ningpoensis (*Yuan Shen*), Bulbus Fritillariae (*Bei Mu*), Spica Prunellae Vulgaris (*Xia Gu Cao*), Herba Sargassii (*Hai Zao*), Thallus Algae (*Kun Bu*), Radix Glycyrrhizae (*Gan Cao*)

Formula explanation: Prepared Radix Rehmanniae and Plastrum Testudinis enrich yin and lie low yang to control vacuous fire. Combining Cortex Phellodendri and Rhizoma Anemarrhenae clears and discharges ministerial fire and protects true yin. Radix Scrophulariae Ningpoensis enriches yin, clears heat, and resolves toxins. Spica Prunellae Vulgaris and Bulbus Fritillariae Thunbergii resolve toxins, transform phlegm, and scatter nodulation. Adding Herba Sargassii and Thallus Algae disperses phlegm and softens the hard. And Radix Glycyrrhizae regulates and harmonizes the preceding medicinals.

Selected acupuncture/moxibustion points: *Tian Jing* (TH 10)⊥, *Shao Hai* (Ht 3)⊥, *Bai Lao* (M-HN-30)⊤, *Shen Shu* (Bl 23)⊤, & *Tai Xi* (Ki 3)⊤

Formula rationale: *Shao Hai* is the sea point of the hand *shao yin*. It downbears heart fire and transforms phlegm turbidity. Combined with *Tian Jing*, it forms an empirical formula for the treatment of scrofula. *Bai Lao* is an extra-channel point. Supplementing it treats scrofula. Supplementing *Shen Shu* enriches and supplements kidney yin. *Tai Xi* is the source point of the kidney channel. Supplementing it enriches yin and downbears fire.

3. *Tan Yu Hu Zu*
Phlegm & (Blood) Stasis Mutually Obstructing

Clinical manifestations: Scrofula all over, firm and hard, immovable when pushed, adhesions becoming lumps or soreness and pain securing, congealing, and becoming immovable, a dark purplish tongue, and a wiry, choppy pulse

Treatment principles: Transform phlegm and resolve toxins, soften the hard and scatter nodulation

Guiding formula: *Xi Huang Wan Jia Jian*

Medicinals: Resina Olibani (*Ru Xiang*), Resina Myrrhae (*Mo Yao*), Calculus Bovis Syntheticus (*Xi Huang*), Secretio Moschi Moschiferi (*She Xiang*), Radix Scrophulariae Ningpoensis (*Yuan Shen*), Spica Prunellae Vulgaris (*Xia Gu Cao*), Bulbus Fritillariae (*Bei Mu*), Radix Ranunculi Ternatae (*Mao Gua Cao*), Rhizoma Dioscoreae Bulbiferae (*Huang Yao Zi*), ginger-processed Rhizoma Pinelliae Ternatae (*Jiang Ban Xia*), Concha Ostreae (*Sheng Mu Li*), Radix Paridis Polyphyllae (*Zai Xiu*), processed Rhizoma Arisaematis (*Zhi Nan Xing*)

Formula explanation: In this formula, man-made Calculus Bovis and Secretio Moschi Moschiferi combined together are the ruling medicinals and clear heat and resolve toxins, quicken the blood and scatter nodulation. Resina Olibani and Resina Myrrhae quicken the blood and transform stasis. Radix Scrophulariae Ningpoensis resolves toxins and scatters nodulation. Spica Prunellae Vulgaris and Bulbus Fritillariae clear heat, transform phlegm, and scatter nodulation. Radix Ranunculi Ternatae and Rhizoma Dioscoreae Bulbiferae clear heat and resolve toxins, scatter nodulation and disperse scrofula. Concha Ostreae softens the hard and scatters nodulation. Radix Paridis Polyphyllae resolves toxins and disperses swelling. Rhizoma Praeparatus Arisaematis and Rhizoma Pinelliae Ternatae transform phlegm and soften the hard. Used together, these medicinals have the ability to transform phlegm and resolve toxins, disperse stasis and scatter scrofula.

Selected acupuncture/moxibustion points: *Tian Jing* (TH 10)⊥, *Qu Chi* (LI 11)⊥, *Feng Long* (St 40)⊥, & *Ge Shu* (Bl 17)⊥

Formula rationale: *Tian Jing* is chosen to disperse scrofula. Draining *Qu Chi* resolves toxins and disperses swelling. *Feng Long* transforms phlegm and scatters nodulation. And draining *Ge Shu*, the meeting point of the blood, eliminates stasis and frees the network vessels, regulates the qi and scatters nodulation.

4. *Qi Xue Kui Xu*
Qi & Blood Deficient & Vacuous

Clinical manifestations: Swelling and kernels in the neck, lack of strength in the four limbs, a pale white facial complexion, dizziness, blurred vision, emaciation, lassitude of the spirit, food and drink not downbearing, shortness of breath on moving, a thin, slimy tongue fur, and a fine, forceless pulse

Treatment principles: Greatly supplement the qi and blood, transform phlegm and scatter nodulation

Guiding formula: *Xiang Bei Yang Ying Wan Jia Jian*

Medicinals: Prepared Radix Rehmanniae (*Shu Di*), Radix Angelicae Sinensis (*Dang Gui*), Radix Albus Paeoniae Lactiflorae (*Bai Shao*), Radix Ligustici Wallichii (*Chuan Xiong*), Radix Panacis Ginseng (*Ren Shen*), Rhizoma Atractylodis Macrocephalae (*Bai Zhu*), Sclerotium Poriae Cocos (*Fu Ling*), Radix Praeparatus Glycyrrhizae (*Zhi Gan Cao*), Rhizoma Cyperi Rotundi (*Xiang Fu*), Bulbus Fritillariae (*Bei Mu*), Rhizoma Dioscoreae Bulbiferae (*Huang Yao Zi*), Radix Semiaguilegiae (*Tian Kui Zi*), calcined Concha Ostreae (*Duan Mu Li*), Pericarpium Citri Reticulatae (*Chen Pi*), uncooked Rhizoma Zingiberis (*Sheng Jiang*), Fructus Zizyphi Jujubae (*Da Zao*)

Formula explanation: In this formula, *Si Jun Zi Tang* supplements the middle and boosts the qi. *Si Wu Tang* supplements and engenders the blood. Together they supplement both qi and blood and are effective for treating qi and blood vacuity. Rhizoma Cyperi Rotundi and Pericarpium Citri Reticulatae move the qi and transform phlegm. If the qi moves, phlegm is dispersed. Concha Ostreae and Bulbus Fritillariae transform phlegm, soften the hard, and scatter nodulation. Rhizoma Dioscoreae Bulbiferae and Radix Semiaquilegiae resolve toxins and scatter nodulation. Fructus Zizyphi Jujubae and uncooked Rhizoma Zingiberis regulate and harmonize the constructive and defensive to treat vacuity.

Note: During the course of treatment, patients may also take internally the Chinese patient medicine *Xiao Jin Dan* twice per day, 1 pill morning and evening, to strengthen the functions of transforming stasis and scattering nodulation.

Selected acupuncture/moxibustion points: *Tian Jing* (Th 10)⊥, *Bai Lao* (M-HN-30)⊤, *Zu San Li* (St 36)⊤x, & *Da Zhui* (Gv 14)|

Formula rationale: *Bai Lao* is an extra-channel point. Supplementing it treats vacuous taxation and disperses scrofula. *Tian Jing* is chosen as an empirical point. Needling and then moxaing *Zu San Li* cultivates and supplements the postnatal, supplements and boosts qi and blood. And even supplementation and drainage of *Da Zhui* aids yang and expels evil. Used together, these points support the righteous, eliminate evil, and scatter nodulation.

X. *Yan Tong*
Sore Throat

Sore throat in AIDS is a commonly seen symptom of opportunistic infection. Usually sore throat is caused by inflammation or ulceration of the throat or tonsils in turn often caused by *Staphylococcus, Streptococcus, Pseudomonas aeruginosa*, or candidal infection of the nasopharynx, the back of the throat, epiglottis, and vocal chords resulting in difficulty speaking. Additionally, overstrain of the digestive tract may lead to inflammation and hence signs of throat pain and difficulty swallowing.

A. Disease Causes, Disease Mechanisms

This disease is caused by none other than righteous qi deficiency and vacuity aggravated by the invasion of wind heat toxic evils. These enter through the mouth and nose and the throat and larynx are the first to be affected. Evil toxins wrestle and knot in the tonsils, blocking and obstructing the vessels and network vessels and giving rise to hot, red, swollen, distended, and painful tonsils. If the evils intrude further internally, going from the exterior to the interior, lung and stomach heat backs up. Toxic evils wrestle and knot above, therefore causing stasis and stagnation of qi and blood in the throat and larynx. The flesh and membranes there are burnt or scorched causing ulceration and sores in the throat and larynx. Additionally, if lung yin is deficient and vacuous and fluids and humors insufficient, they are incapable of transporting upwards and enriching and nourishing the throat and larynx. In that case, there will be vacuous yin and internal heat. Vacuous fire then flames upwards. This may also cause sore throat.

B. Differentiation & Treatment

1. *Xie Re Wai Dai*
Evil Heat (in) the Outer Pockets, *i.e.*, Tonsils

Clinical manifestations: Sore throat gradually getting more severe, a dry throat which feels burning hot, red, swollen ulcers in the throat and larynx usually accompanied by fever, bodily fatigue, cough, a red tongue tip and sides, thin, white or slightly yellow fur, and a floating, rapid pulse

Treatment principles: Course the wind and clear heat, disperse swelling and disinhibit the throat

Guiding formula: *Shu Feng Qing Re Tang Jia Jian*

Medicinals: Flos Lonicerae Japonicae (*Yin Hua*), Fructus Forsythiae Suspensae (*Lian Qiao*), Fructus Arctii Lappae (*Niu Bang Zi*), Cortex Radicis Mori Albi (*Sang Bai Pi*), Radix Rubrus Paeoniae Lactiflorae (*Chi Shao*), Radix Scutellariae Baicalensis (*Huang Qin*), Radix Platycodi Grandiflori (*Jie Geng*), Radix Trichosanthis Kirlowii (*Hua Fen*), Radix Scrophulariae Ningpoensis (*Yuan Shen*), Bulbus Fritillariae Cirrhosae (*Chuan Bei Mu*), Radix Glycyrrhizae (*Gan Cao*)

Formula explanation: In this formula, Flos Lonicerae Japonicae and Fructus Forsythiae Suspensae course wind, clear heat, and relieve the exterior. Radix Scutellariae Baicalensis clears and discharges lung heat. Fructus Arctii Lappae and Radix Platycodi Grandiflori resolve toxins and disinhibit the throat. Radix Rubrus Paeoniae Lactiflorae clears heat and cools the blood. Cortex Radicis Mori Albi and Bulbus Fritillariae Cirrhosae clear the lungs and transform phlegm. Radix Scrophulariae Ningpoensis and Radix Trichosanthis Kirlowii clear heat and engender fluids. Radix Glycyrrhizae regulates and harmonizes the preceding medicinals.

Selected acupuncture/moxibustion points: *Da Zhui* (GV 14)|, *Qu Chi* (LI 11)⊥, *He Gu* (LI 4)⊥, *Shao Shang* (Lu 11)↓, & *Lie Que* (Lu 7)⊥

Formula rationale: *Da Zhui* aids yang, relieves the exterior, and expels evil. Draining *Qu Chi* clears heat and resolves toxins. Bleeding *Shao Shang* discharges lung heat and disperses swelling and pain. Draining *He Gu* clears heat and relieves the exterior, courses wind, and diffuses the lungs. *Lie Que* clears and discharges lung heat and stops coughing.

2. *Fei Wei Yun Re*
Lungs & Stomach Accumulate Heat

Clinical manifestations: Severe sore throat, throat and larynx red and swollen or ulcerated accompanied by high fever, thirst with desire to drink, a bad taste in the mouth, abdominal distention, scant, yellow urine, a red tongue with yellow fur, and a surging, big, rapid pulse

Treatment principles: Clear heat and resolve toxins, disinhibit the throat and disperse swelling

Guiding formula: *Qing Yan Li Ge Tang Jia Jian*

Medicinals: Fructus Forsythiae Suspensae (*Lian Qiao*), Fructus Gardeniae Jasminoidis (*Zhi Zi*), Radix Scutellariae Baicalensis (*Huang Qin*), Fructus Arctii Lappae (*Niu Bang Zi*), Herba Menthae Haplocalycis (*Bo He*), Radix Ledebouriellae Sesloidis (*Fang Feng*), Radix Scrophulariae Ningpoensis (*Yuan Shen*), Flos Lonicerae Japonicae (*Yin Hua*), Radix Et Rhizoma Rhei (*Da Huang*)

Formula explanation: In this formula, Fructus Gardeniae Jasminoidis and Radix Scutellariae Baicalensis clear heat and resolve toxins. Fructus Forsythiae Suspensae and Flos Lonicerae Japonicae combined with Fructus Gardeniae Jasminoidis and Radix Scutellariae Baicalensis have a strong ability to drain fire and resolve toxins. Radix Scrophulariae Ningpoensis and Fructus Arctii Lappae resolve toxins and disinhibit the throat. Herba Menthae Haplocalycis and Radix Ledebouriellae Sesloidis clear and course wind and scatter evils. Radix Et Rhizoma Rhei is chosen to free the bowels and discharge heat or, in other words, purge heat downwards.

Selected acupuncture/moxibustion points: *Shang Yang* (St 45)↓, *Nei Ting* (St 44)⊥, *Qu Chi* (LI 11)⊥, *Tian Tu* (CV 22)⊥, & *Feng Long* (St 40)⊥

Formula rationale: Bleeding the well point of the hand *yang ming* channel, *Shang Yang*, is chosen to discharge heat and stop pain. Draining the spring point of the foot *yang ming* channel clears heat accumulated in the *yang ming*. *Qu Chi* clears heat, resolves toxins, and disperses swelling. *Tian Tu* is the meeting point of the *yin wei* and *ren* *mai*. Therefore it clears and disinhibits the throat. Draining *Feng Long* clears heat, transforms phlegm, and disinhibits the portals.

3. *Fei Shen Yin Xu*
Lung/Kidney Yin Vacuity

Clinical manifestations: Chronic sore, painful throat, repeated occurrence accompanied by tidal fever, night sweats, cheeks red, dry mouth and throat, mind weary and tired, hands, feet, heart hot, a red tongue with scant fur, and a fine, rapid pulse

Treatment principles: Nourish yin and clear heat, engender fluids and moisten dryness

Guiding formula: *Bai He Gu Jin Tang Jia Jian*

Medicinals: Uncooked Radix Rehmanniae (*Sheng Di*), prepared Radix Rehmanniae (*Shu Di*), Tuber Ophiopogonis Japonicae (*Mai Dong*), Bulbus Fritillariae Cirrhosae (*Chuan Bei Mu*), Bulbus Lilii (*Bai He*), Radix Angelicae Sinensis (*Dang Gui*), Radix Scrophulariae Ningpoensis (*Yuan Shen*), Radix Platycodi Grandiflori (*Jie Geng*), Radix Albus Paeoniae Lactiflorae (*Bai Shao*), Cortex Radicis Moutan (*Dan Pi*), Radix Glycyrrhizae (*Gan Cao*)

Formula explanation: Uncooked Radix Rehmanniae clears heat and nourishes yin. Prepared Radix Rehmanniae enriches and supplements kidney yin. Tuber Ophiopogonis Japonicae and Bulbus Lilii nourish yin and moisten the lungs to clear heat. Radix Angelicae Sinensis and Radix Albus Paeoniae Lactiflorae restrain yin and nourish the blood. Bulbus Fritillariae Cirrhosae clears the lungs and transforms phlegm. Radix Scrophulariae Ningpoensis and Radix Platycodi Grandiflori resolve toxins and disinhibit the throat. Cortex Radicis Moutan cools the blood and recedes heat or fever. Radix Glycyrrhizae resolves toxins and regulates and harmonizes the preceding medicinals.

If accompanied by shortness of breath and lack of strength, food consumption reduced, weary and unable to work, disinclination to speak, a pale tongue with thin fur, a fine, forceless pulse, and other signs of qi vacuity, add Radix Codonopsis Pilosulae (*Dang Shen*), Radix Astragali Membranacei (*Huang Qi*), Rhizoma Atractylodis Macrocephalae (*Bai Zhu*), and Radix Dioscoreae Oppositae (*Shan Yao*) to the above formula to boost the qi.

Selected acupuncture/moxibustion points: *Tai Xi* (Ki 3)⊥, *Zhao Hai* (Ki 6)|, *Yu Ji* (Lu 10)⊥, & *Ye Men* (TH 2)|

Formula rationale: *Tai Xi* is the foot *shao yin* source point. Supplementing it is able to enrich and supplement kidney yin. *Zhao Hai* is one of the meeting points of the eight vessels. It frees the throat and larynx. Draining it enriches yin and clears heat, disinhibits the throat and stops pain. *Yu Ji* is the spring point of the lung channel. Draining it clears lung heat, disinhibits the throat and larynx. Even supplementation and drainage of *Ye Men* engenders fluids and moistens dryness.

XI. *Kou Chuang*
Oral Apathae, *i.e.*, Thrush

In full blown AIDS, many patients have thrush and stomatitis. Because of patient's hypoimmunity, there are repeated infections of the oral cavity. The causes of these infections are Herpes simplex virus, *Candida albicans, Staphylococcus, Streptococcus, Cryptosporidia*, and Cytomegalovirus. The most commonly seen are fungal infections. Since these fungus often stimulate the oral mucosa, there are usually leukoplakia. And in thrush, there is a layer of white curdy material covering the oral cavity and membranes.

A. Disease Causes, Disease Mechanisms

This disease usually manifests due to righteous qi deficiency and vacuity and lowering of the body's disease resistance plus retention of evil toxins due to vacuity. These evil toxins accumulate and stagnate in the spleen and stomach. Depression transforms into fire and flares upward to steam and scorch the oral cavity. This corrupts the flesh and membranes causing ulceration of the mucosa and pain or covering the oral cavity with a white, curdy material. Or, if kidney yin is deficient and vacuous, water cannot control fire and vacuous fire floats upward. If evil toxins have also invaded internally, this may result in apthae or thrush. This condition may also be caused by spleen/stomach middle qi suffering detriment with spleen/stomach qi vacuity. Yin fire arises internally causing thrush.

B. Differentiation & Treatment

1. *Xin Pi Ji Re*
Heart/Spleen Accumulation of Heat

Clinical manifestations: Ulceration of the lips, tongue, and mouth with red, swollen borders or white curds filling the oral cavity, thirst with a desire to drink, body feels hot, yellowish-red urine, a red tongue with yellow fur, and a rapid pulse.

Treatment principles: Clear heat and discharge fire

Guiding formula: *Liang Ge San Jia Jian*

Medicinals: Radix Scutellariae Baicalensis (*Huang Qin*), Rhizoma Coptidis Chinensis (*Huang Lian*), Fructus Gardeniae Jasminoidis (*Zhi Zi*), uncooked Radix Rehmanniae (*Sheng Di*), Tuber Ophiopogonis Japonicae (*Mai Dong*), Herba Lophatheri Gracilis (*Zhu Ye*), Herba Menthae Haplocalycis (*Bo He*), Radix Glycyrrhizae (*Sheng Gan Cao*)

Formula explanation: Radix Scutellariae Baicalensis, Rhizoma Coptidis Chinensis, and Fructus Gardeniae Jasminoidis clear heat, resolve toxins, and drain fire. Herba Lophatheri Gracilis clears heat, eliminates vexation, and engenders fluids. Herba Menthae Haplocalycis lightly clears and courses the exterior and guides the other medicinals upwards. Uncooked Radix Rehmanniae and Tuber Ophiopogonis Japonicae enrich yin and clear heat, engender fluids and stop thirst. Radix Glycyrrhizae resolves toxins and also regulates and harmonizes the preceding medicinals.

Selected acupuncture/moxibustion points: *He Gu* (LI 4)⊥, *Qu Chi* (LI 11)⊥, *Feng Long* (St 40)⊥, *Lao Gong* (Per 8)⊥, & *Shao Ze* (SI 1)↓

Formula ratonale: The spring point of the pericardium channel, *Lao Gong*, is chosen to clear heart fire and resolve toxins. This point effectively treats thrush. Bleeding *Shao Ze* clears the heart, eliminates vexation, and stops pain. Draining *He Gu* and *Qu Chi* clears *yang ming* channel heat, courses the exterior, and resolves toxins. Draining *Feng Long* transforms phlegm and drains internally accumulated heat.

2. *Xu Huo Shang Yan*
Vacuous Fire Flares Upward

Clinical manifestations: Sparse, scattered white curds in the mouth or ulceration of the mouth and tongue, soreness and pain which is more severe at night than during the day, a dry mouth, hands, feet, and heart hot, heart vexation, loss of sleep, a red tongue with scant fur, and a fine, rapid pulse

Treatment principles: Enrich yin and downbear fire

Guiding formula: *Zhi Bai Di Huang Wan Jia Jian*

Medicinals: Cortex Phellodendri (*Huang Bai*), Rhizoma Anemarrhenae (*Zhi Mu*), prepared Radix Rehmanniae (*Shu Di*), Cortex Radicis Moutan (*Dan Pi*), Rhizoma Alismatis (*Ze Xie*), Sclerotium Poriae Cocos

(*Fu Ling*), Tuber Ophiopogonis Japonicae (*Mai Dong*), Fructus Schizandrae Chinensis (*Wu Wei Zi*)

Formula explanation: Cortex Phellodendri and Rhizoma Anemarrhenae clear heat, resolve toxins, and drain vacuous fire. Prepared Radix Rehmanniae enriches yin and supplements the kidneys. Cortex Radicis Moutan and Rhizoma Alismatis drain, clear, and discharge kidney fire to resolve toxins and cool the blood. Sclerotium Poriae Cocos blandly seeps and disinhibits dampness. Tuber Ophiopogonis Japonicae and Fructus Schizandrae Chinensis enrich yin and clear heat, engender fluids and eliminate vexation.

Selected acupuncture/moxibustion points: *Tai Xi* (Ki 3)⊤, *Lao Gong* (Per 8)⊥, & *Zhao Hai* (Ki 6)⊥

Formula rationale: Supplementing *Tai Xi* enriches and supplements kidney yin and downbears vacuous fire. Draining *Lao Gong* clears the heart and drains fire, cools the blood and eliminates vexation. It is also good for treating thrush. Draining *Zhao Hai* clears and discharges kidney fire and enriches kidney water.

3. *Zhong Qi Bu Zu*
Center Qi Insufficiency

Clinical manifestations: Repeated apthae, sometimes light, sometimes severe, lesions light colored, reduced appetite, epigastric distention, loose stools or diarrhea, extremities weak, lassitude of the spirit, shortness of breath, disinclination to speak, a pale tongue with white fur, and a weak pulse

Treatment principles: Supplement the center and boost the qi assisted by resolving toxins

Guiding formula: *Bu Zhong Yi Qi Tang Jia Jian*

Medicinals: Radix Astragali Membranacei (*Huang Qi*), Radix Codonopsis Pilosulae (*Dang Shen*), Rhizoma Atractylodis Macrocephalae (*Bai Zhu*), Radix Angelicae Sinensis (*Dang Gui*), Pericarpium Citri Reticulatae (*Chen Pi*), Rhizoma Cimicifugae (*Sheng Ma*), Radix Bupleuri (*Chai Hu*), Rhizoma Coptidis Chinensis (*Huang Lian*), Herba Lophatheri Gracilis (*Zhu Ye*), Radix Glycyrrhizae (*Gan Cao*)

Formula explanation: In this formula, Radix Astragali Membranacei supplements the center and boosts the qi. It is assisted by the combination of Radix Codonopsis Pilosulae and Rhizoma Atractylodis Macrocephalae which boosts the qi and fortifies the spleen. Pericarpium Citri Reticulatae regulates the qi and harmonizes the stomach. Radix Angelicae Sinensis nourishes the blood. Adding a little Rhizoma Cimicifugae and Radix Bupleuri aids the ruling medicinals in upbearing the prolapse of yang qi. Adding Rhizoma Coptidis Chinensis and Herba Lophatheri Gracilis clears heat and resolves toxins. Radix Glycyrrhizae regulates and harmonizes the preceding medicinals.

Note: Various medicines, such as *Bing Peng San, Xi Lei San*, and *Zhu Huang San*, can be applied externally for this condition.

Selected acupuncture/moxibustion points: *Zu San Li* (St 36)⊥, *Zhong Wan* (CV 12)⊥, *Qi Hai* (CV 6)⊥▲, & *Lao Gong* (Per 8)|

Formula rationale: Supplementing *Zu San Li* boosts the qi and engenders blood, fortifies the spleen and boosts the stomach. Supplementing *Zhong Wan* aids transportation to disperse distention and fullness. Needling and then moxaing *Qi Hai* supplements the source qi, warms the yang, and boosts the qi. Even supplementation and drainage of *Lao Gong* clears the heart and resolves toxins. Used together, these points supplement the center and boosts the qi, thus dispelling this pathocondition.

XII. *Pao Zhen*
Herpes

Various skin diseases typically occur as a result of the decline in immunity associated with AIDS. Herpes is usually caused by invasion of the virus into the skin cells, thus leading to the formation of water blisters. Herpes simplex usually causes clusters of small, watery blisters around the genital organs or anus accompanied by slight itching. Herpes zoster usually causes clusters of blisters with red, swollen borders distributed along the peripheral nerves in the form of stripes. This is commonly accompanied by fever, aching and pain, or local swelling of the lymph nodes. In the later stages of AIDS, there may also be malignant tumors. This disease can often be very severe, causing bleeding, necrosis, and post-herpetic neuralgia.

A. Disease Causes, Disease Mechanisms

Herpes simplex is categorized in TCM as *re chuang* or "hot ulcers" and herpes zoster is called in TCM *she cuan chuang* or "snake-like ulcers". The disease cause is usually righteous qi vacuity with wind and fire evils invading internally taking advantage of vacuity. These may further accumulate in the *shao yin* and *jue yin* channels and occlude the skin causing damp toxic evils to accumulate internally. This steams the flesh and skin resulting in qi and blood obstruction and stagnation. If damp heat pours downward, this can cause herpes in the genitalia.

B. Differentiation & Treatment

1. *Gan Jing Feng Huo*
Liver Channel Wind & Fire

Clinical manifestations: Skin flushed red, clusters of blisters with burning heat and stabbing pain, a bitter taste in the mouth and dry throat, thirst, scant, red urine, vexation and agitation, easily angered, a red tongue with yellow fur, and a wiry, rapid pulse

Treatment principles: Drain liver/gallbladder replete fire, simultaneously clear heat and disinhibit dampness

Guiding formula: *Long Dan Xie Gan Tang Jia Jian*

Medicinals: Radix Gentianae Scabrae (*Long Dan Cao*), Radix Scutellariae Baicalensis (*Huang Qin*), Fructus Gardeniae Jasminoidis (*Shan Zhi*), Rhizoma Alismatis (*Ze Xie*), Caulis Akebiae (*Mu Tong*), Semen Plantaginis (*Che Qian Zi*), Radix Bupleuri (*Chai Hu*), uncooked Radix Rehmanniae (*Sheng Di*), Radix Angelicae Sinensis (*Dang Gui*), Radix Glycyrrhizae (*Gan Cao*)

Radix Scutellariae Baicalensis and Fructus Gardeniae Jasmino **Formula explanation:** In this formula, Radix Gentianae Scabrae drains liver/gallbladder replete heat and eliminates damp heat from the lower burner. idis, bitter and cold, clear heat and resolve toxins. Radix Bupleuri courses the liver and resolves depression to recede heat. Caulis Akebiae, Rhizoma Alismatis, and Semen Plantaginis clear and disinhibit damp heat and guide out fire via urination. Radix Angelicae Sinensis nourishes and activates the blood. Uncooked Radix Rehmanniae clears heat and engenders fluids. And Radix Glycyrrhizae regulates and harmonizes the preceding medicinals.

Selected acupuncture/moxibustion points: Needle (local points) surrounding the affected area, *Qi Men* (Liv 14)|, *Yang Ling Quan* (GB 34)⊥, *Zu Qiao Yin* (GB 44)⊥, & *Nei Ting* (St 44)⊥

Formula rationale: Local points surrounding the affected area are needled to quicken the blood, disperse inflammation, and stop pain. *Qi Men* courses the liver and resolves depression. *Yang Ling Quan* is the sea point of the gallbladder channel. It courses and discharges liver/gallbladder depressive fire. *Zu Qiao Yin* courses and scatters *shao yang* evils. *Nei Ting* is the spring point of the foot *yang ming*. Draining it clears and disinhibits damp heat.

2. *Shi Du Yun Jie*
Damp Toxins Accumulate & Bind

Clinical manifestations: The eruption of herpes lesions on the skin with ulcers and exudation, exhaustion, fatigue, lack of strength, thirst with no desire to drink, extremities and body tired and weary, poor appetite, loose stools, a pale tongue with yellow, slimy fur, and a soggy, rapid pulse

Treatment principles: Fortify the spleen and disinhibit dampness, simultaneously clear heat and resolve toxins

Guiding formula: *Wei Ling Tang Jia Jian*

Medicinals: Sclerotium Poriae Cocos (*Fu Ling*), Sclerotium Polpori Umbellati (*Zhu Ling*), Rhizoma Alsimatis (*Ze Xie*), Talcum (*Hua Shi*), Fructus Gardeniae Jasminoidis (*Zhi Zi*), Caulis Akebiae (*Mu Tong*), Rhizoma Atractylodis (*Cang Zhu*), Cortex Magnoliae Officinalis (*Hou Po*), Pericarpium Citri Reticulatae (*Chen Pi*), Medulla Junci Effusi (*Deng Xin Cao*), Radix Glycyrrhizae (*Gan Cao*)

Formula explanation: Sclerotium Poriae Cocos blandly seeps, disinhibits dampness, and fortifies the spleen. Sclerotium Polpori Umbellati, Rhizoma Alismatis, and Talcum disinhibit water and seep dampness. Rhizoma Atractylodis and Cortex Magnoliae Officinalis dry dampness and fortify the spleen. Caulis Akebiae and Medulla Junci Effusi clear heat and disinhibit dampness, lead heat down and move (it out). Pericparpium Citri Reticulatae regulates the qi, dries dampness, and harmonizes the middle. Radix Glycyrrhizae regulates and harmonizes the preceding medicinals.

Note: For blisters which are not broken, apply *Shuang Bai San* or *Jin Huang San* externally. For those already broken, apply *Si Huang Gao* or *Qing Dai Gao* externally.

Selected acupuncture/moxibustion points: Needle local points surrounding the affected area, *Tai Chong* (Liv 3)⊥, *Gong Sun* (Sp 4)⊥, *Yin Ling Quan* (Sp 9)⊥, & *Xue Hai* (Sp 10)⊥

Formula rationale: Draining *Tai Chong* clears and discharges liver/gallbladder heat. *Gong Sun* is the network point of the spleen channel. Draining it clears and disinhibits damp heat. *Yin Ling Quan* is the sea point. Draining it fortifies the spleen and disinhibits dampness. Draining *Xue Hai* clears stagnant heat from the blood aspect and resolves toxins.

Note: Disinfect the local area first. Then bleed the head and tail of the herpes stripe. Next puncture several needles subcutaneously towards the center line of the herpes. Retain the needles for 30-60 minutes. Needle 1-2 times per day.

XIII. *Sao Yang* Pruritus

Sao Yang, literally scratching and itching, is an unpleasant sensation in the skin resulting from various harms to the skin. It is a commonly seen condition in AIDS patients suffering from opportunistic infections. Those with seborrheic dermatitis usually have reddish spots or scaling on the face or dandruff. Skin rashes are usually diffuse, nonspecific maculopapulae which are caused by mycotic infection of the skin. In addition, there may also be cases of fungal infection of the skin or even the fingernails, eczema, etc. all of which may cause outbreaks of scratching and itching.

A. Disease Causes, Disease Mechanisms

The causes of this disease are usually very complicated and the disease mechanisms are extremely variable. The internal causes are mostly qi and blood deficiency and vacuity with loss of regulation of the viscera and bowel qi mechanism and that of yin and yang. The external causes are mostly wind evils taking advantage of vacuity and invading the exterior. Deficiency and vacuity of qi and blood may cause the defensive exterior to be unsecured. Hence wind evils may invade externally. Meanwhile, blood heat may arise internally causing transformative dryness. The flesh and skin lose their nourishment and thus the itching.

Vacuity of qi and blood may cause vacuity of blood production or damp toxic evils may accumulate internally. Further, the exterior may suffer from wind heat, damp and heat evils may mutually wrestle and knot, or excessive, licentious immersion of the skin may cause the skin to itch.

B. Differentiation & Treatment

1. *Xue Re Feng Zao*
Blood Heat, Wind Dryness

Clinical manifestations: Skin flushed or weals and rashes, dry skin, scratching and itching, desquamation, bleeding due to scratching and breaking the skin, a red tongue with thin, white fur, and a wiry, slippery pulse

Treatment principles: Cool the blood and clear heat, disperse wind and moisten dryness

Guiding formula: *Xiao Feng San Jia Jian*

Medicinals: Herba Schizonepetae Tenuifoliae (*Jing Jie*), Radix Ledebouriellae Sesloidis (*Fang Feng*), Radix Angelicae Sinensis (*Dang Gui*), uncooked Radix Rehmanniae (*Sheng Di*), Radix Sophorae Flavescentis (*Ku Shen*), Rhizoma Atractylodis (*Cang Zhu*), Periostracum Cicadae (*Chan Tui*), Semen Sesami Indici (*Hu Ma Ren*), Fructus Arctii Lappae (*Niu Bang Zi*), Rhizoma Anemarrhenae (*Zhi Mu*), Gypsum Fibrosum (*Shi Gao*), Radix Glycyrrhizae (*Gan Cao*)

Formula explanation: Herba Schizonepetae Tenuifoliae, Radix Ledebouriellae Sesloidis, Periostracum Cicadae, and Fructus Arctii Lapae out-thrust the exterior, course wind, and stop itching. Rhizoma Atractylodis scatters wind and eliminates dampness. Radix Sophorae Flavescentis clears heat and dries dampness. Caulis Akebiae seeps and disinhibits damp heat. Gypsum Fibrosum and Rhizoma Anemarrhenae clear heat and drain fire. Radix Angelicae Sinensis harmonizes the constructive and activates the blood. Uncooked Radix Rehmanniae clears heat and cools the blood. Semen Sesami Indici nourishes the blood and moistens dryness. And Radix Glycyrrhizae regulates and harmonizes the preceding medicinals while simultaneously resolving toxins.

Selected acupuncture/moxibustion points: *Da Zhui* (GV 14)⊥, *He Gu* (LI 4)⊥, *Feng Chi* (GB 20)⊥, *Xue Hai* (Sp 10)⊥, & *Shen Men* (Ht 7)⊥

Formula rationale: Draining *Da Zhui* courses and scatters wind heat, aids yang and expels evil. Draining *He Gu* clears heat from the qi aspect, courses wind, and stops itching. Draining *Feng Chi* courses wind and clears heat. Draining *Shen Men* clears the heart, tranquilizes the heart, quiets the spirit, and stops itching. Draining *Xue Hai* clears heat from the blood aspect, drains the blood and harmonizes the constructive.

2. *Pi Wei Shi Re*
Spleen/Stomach Damp Heat

Clinical manifestations: Itching of the skin, weals and rashes, water blisters after scratching, exudation or extremely wet skin ulcers, dry mouth, yellow urine, a red tongue with yellow, slimy fur

Treatment principles: Disinhibit dampness and clear heat, disperse wind and stop itching

Guiding formula: *Long Dan Xie Gan Tang Jia Jian*

Medicinals: Radix Gentianae Scabrae (*Long Dan Cao*), Fructus Gardeniae Jasminoidis (*Zhi Zi*), Radix Scutellariae Baicalensis (*Huang Qin*), Radix Bupleuri (*Chai Hu*), Semen Plantaginis (*Che Qian Zi*), uncooked Radix Rehmanniae (*Sheng Di*), Rhizoma Alismatis (*Ze Xie*), Caulis Akebiae (*Mu Tong*), Radix Ledebouriellae Sesloidis (*Fang Feng*), Radix Glycyrrhizae (*Gan Cao*)

Formula explanation: Radix Gentianae Scabrae is chosen to clear and disinhibit damp heat in the lower burner. Radix Scutellariae Baicalensis and Fructus Gardeniae Jasminoidis, bitter and cold, drain fire and resolve toxins. Radix Bupleuri courses the liver and resolves depression.

Semen Plantaginis, Rhizoma Alismatis, and Caulis Akebiae clear heat and disinhibit dampness, guide heat evils out via urination. Uncooked Radix Rehmanniae clears heat and engenders fluids. Adding Radix Ledebouriellae Sesloidis courses and scatters wind evils. Used together, these medicinals disinhibit dampness and clear heat, disperse wind and stop itching.

Selected acupuncture/moxibustion points: *Qu Chi* (LI 11)⊥, *Zu San Li* (St 36)⊥, *Xue Hai* (Sp 10)⊥, & *Yin Ling Quan* (Sp 9)⊥

Formula rationale: Choosing the sea points of the hand and foot *yang ming* channel, *Qu Chi* and *Zu San Li*, clears and discharges stagnant heat from the *yang ming*. Draining *Xue Hai* in combination with *Yin Ling Quan* clears heat, disinhibits dampness, and stops itching. When the above points are used together, they eliminate damp heat and thus automatically relieve this pathocondition.

3. *Xue Xu Feng Zao*
Blood Vacuity, Wind Dryness

Clinical manifestations: Dry skin full of scratches, desquamation or bleeding, itching sometimes during the day, sometimes at night accompanied by a lustreless facial complexion, heart palpitations, loss of sleep, dizziness, blurred vision, a red tongue with thin fur, and a wiry, fine pulse

Treatment principles: Boost the qi and nourish the blood, expel wind and stop itching

Guiding formula: *Dang Gui Yin Zi Jia Jian*

Medicinals: Radix Angelicae Sinensis (*Dang Gui*), Radix Albus Paeoniae Lactiflorae (*Bai Shao*), Radix Ligustici Wallichii (*Chuan Xiong*), uncooked Radix Rehmanniae (*Sheng Di*), Fructus Tribuli Terrestris (*Bai Ji Li*), Herba Schizonepetae Tenuifoliae (*Jing Jie*), Radix Ledebouriellae Sesloidis (*Fang Feng*), Radix Polygoni Multiflori (*He*

163

Shou Wu), Radix Astragali Membranacei (*Huang Qi*), Radix Glycyrrhizae (*Gan Cao*)

Formula explanation: In this formula, *Si Wu Tang* boosts and regulates the blood, nourishes the blood and harmonizes the constructive. Herba Schizonepetae Tenuifoliae and Radix Ledebouriellae Sesloidis course external evils, disperse wind, and stop itching. Radix Polygoni Multiflori nourishes and engenders blood. Radix Astragali Membranacei supplements the qi. Fructus Tribuli Terrestris courses the liver and resolves depression, expels wind and stops itching. Radix Glycyrrhizae harmonizes the middle. Used together, these medicinals have the ability to supplement the qi and engender blood, expel wind and stop itching.

Note: For those with itching of the whole body, apply *Ku Shen Jiu* externally. For those with itching and dry skin, apply *Run Ji Gao* externally. And for those with only localized itching, wash the affected parts with *Ku Shen Tang* externally.

Selected acupuncture/moxibustion points: *Xue Hai* (Sp 10)т, *San Yin Jiao* (Sp 6)т, *Fu Liu* (Ki 7)т, & *Ge Shu* (Bl 17)т

Formula rationale: Supplementing *Xue Hai* is chosen to nourish the blood and moisten dryness. Supplementing *Fu Liu* enriches and supplements kidney water and moistens dryness. Supplementing *Ge Shu* supplements and activates the blood, nourishes the blood and harmonizes the constructive. *San Yin Jiao* enriches yin and boosts the qi, nourishes the blood and expels wind. Used together, these points boost the qi and engender blood, expel wind and stop itching.

XIV. *Pi Fu Jie Jie*
Skin Tubercles (Kaposi's Sarcoma)

Kaposi's sarcoma is one of the most commonly seen complications in the full blown AIDS stage. Its skin lesions usually present as tubercles or skin rashes. Their size ranges from 0.4-2.5 cm and are colored bluish purple or reddish brown. The tubercles are usually seen on the legs. They take shape gradually or harden into tubercles. In severe cases, the lower legs may become damaged and injured and there may even be bleeding, cankers, and necrosis. Kaposi's sarcoma can also present on the oral mucosa, the back wall of the throat, in the gastrointestinal tract, and in may other organs and tissues throughout the body. In all cases, this disease is very serious.

A. Disease Causes, Disease Mechanisms

The causes of this disease are primarily deficiency and vacuity of the viscera and bowels, qi and blood with qi stagnation and blood stasis as well as phlegm dampness congelation and stagnation which wrestle together and knot and bind in the skin. If the spleen loses its promotion of transportation, damp turbidity will be engenderd internally. When this congeals and gathers together, it turns into this disease. If qi and blood are deficient and vacuous, blood movement is not smooth and unimpeded. The vessels and network vessels become stopped up and jammed. If phlegm turbidity and stagnant blood mutually wrestle and knot together, this may also lead to the onset of this disease. Further, if phlegm turbidity is not transformed and the internal viscera and bowels and the vessels and network vessels become clogged, blood stasis may wrestle and knot with this throughout the body and in the viscera and bowels. Thus the key cause of this disease is deficiency and vacuity of the righteous qi and the resultant blood stasis and phlegm congelation.

B. Differentiation & Treatment

1. *Qi Zhi Xue Yu*
Qi Stagnation, Blood Stasis

Clinical manifestations: Tubercles all over the lower limbs or in the oral cavity gradually darkening and hardening, skin color not changed, a dark purple tongue with yellow fur, and a slippery pulse

Treatment principles: Quicken the blood and transform stasis, resolve toxins and scatter nodulation

Guiding formula: *Jie Du Hua Yu Wan*

Medicinals: Resina Olibani (*Ru Xiang*), Resina Myrrhae (*Mo Yao*), Radix Salviae Miltiorrhizae (*Dan Shen*), Radix Rubrus Paeoniae Lactiflorae (*Chi Shao*), Fructus Forsythiae Suspensae (*Lian Qiao*), Flos Lonicerae Japonicae (*Yin Hua*), Caulis Milletiae Seu Spatholobi (*Ji Xue Teng*), Cortex Radicis Moutan (*Dan Pi*)

Formula explanation: Resina Olibani and Resina Myrrhae are chosen to quicken the blood and transform stasis, disperse swelling and engender new flesh. Radix Salviae Miltiorrhizae quickens and cools the blood. Flos Lonicerae Japonicae and Fructus Forsythiae Suspensae clear heat and resolve toxins. Radix Rubrus Paeoniae Lactiflorae and Cortex Radicis Moutan clear heat and cool the blood, expel stasis and scatter nodulation. Caulis Milletiae Seu Spatholobi quickens and supplements the blood. Used together, these medicinals have the ability to quicken the blood and transform stasis, resolve toxins and scatter nodulation.

Selected acupuncture/moxibustion points: *Zu San Li* (St 36)⊥, *Ge Shu* (Bl 17)⊥, *Shan Zhong* (CV 17)⊥, *Xue Hai* (Sp 10)⊥, & *Tai Chong* (Liv 3)⊥

Formula rationale: Draining *Zu San Li* rectifies the qi, quickens the blood, and scatters stagnation. *Ge Shu* expels stasis and frees the network vessels, rectifies the qi and scatters nodulation. Draining *Shan Zhong* rectifies the qi and loosens the chest. Draining *Xue Hai* moves the blood and expels stasis, transforms dampness and resolves toxins. *Tai Chong* courses the liver and rectifies the qi. Used together, these points quicken the blood and transform stasis, resolve toxins and scatter nodulation.

2. *Xie Du Nei Yun*
Evil Toxins Accumulate Internally

Clinical manifestations: Large or small tubercles mutually fusing and uniting or even ulceration and necrosis, prolonged course does not heal accompanied by an exhausted spirit, lack of strength, poor appetite, limbs heavy and without strength, edema in the feet, extreme emaciation, a pale tongue with thin, yellow fur, and a deep, fine pulse

Treatment principles: Boost the qi and quicken the blood, transform dampness and resolve toxins

Guiding formula: *Sheng Ma Xiao Du Yin*

Medicinals: Rhizoma Cimicifugae (*Sheng Ma*), Radix Astragali Membranacei (*Huang Qi*), Radix Bupleuri (*Chai Hu*), Radix Angelicae Sinensis (*Dang Gui*), Flos Lonicerae Japonicae (*Yin Hua*), Fructus Forsythiae Suspensae (*Lian Qiao*), Fructus Gardeniae Jasminoidis (*Zhi Zi*), Radix Rubrus Paeoniae Lactiflorae (*Chi Shao*), Caulis Milletiae Seu Spatholobi (*Ji Xue Teng*), Cortex Radicis Moutan (*Dan Pi*), Semen Coicis Lachryma-jobi (*Sheng Yi Ren*), Rhizoma Arisaematis (*Nan Xing*)

Formula explanation: Radix Astragali Membranacei is chosen to supplement the qi, force out toxins, and engender new flesh. Rhizoma Cimicifugae and Radix Bupleuri aid the ruling medicinal to lift prolapse of yang qi. Radix Angelicae Sinensis and Caulis Milletiae Seu Spatholobi nourish and cool the blood. Fructus Gardeniae Jasminoidis and Cortex Radicis Moutan resolve toxins and cool the blood. Flos Lonicerae Japonicae and Fructus Forsythiae Suspensae clear heat and resolve toxins. Radix Rubrus Paeoniae Lactiflorae clears heat, resolves toxins, and transforms stasis. Rhizoma Arisaematis resolves toxins and transforms phlegm. Semen Coicis Lachryma-jobi disinhibits dampness and fortifies the spleen. Used together, these medicinals have the ability to support the righteous and eliminate evil, transform stasis and resolve toxins.

Selected acupuncture/moxibustion points: *Pi Shu* (Bl 20)⊤, *Zhong Wan* (CV 12)⊤, *Zu San Li* (St 36)⊥, *Da Zhui* (GV 14)⊤, *Feng Long* (St 40)⊤, & *Yin Ling Quan* (Sp 9)⊥

Formula rationale: Supplementing *Zhong Wan* and *Pi Shu* is chosen to fortify the spleen and boost the stomach, supplement and boost the postnatal. If the spleen is strengthened, damp turbidity will be removed. Draining *Zu San Li* quickens the blood and scatters stasis. Supplementing *Da Zhui* aids yang and expels evil. *Feng Long* transforms phlegm and scatters nodulation. Draining *Yin Ling Quan* fortifies the spleen, transforms dampness, and resolves toxins.

XV. *Shi Wu Hun Meng*
Visual Objects Dim & Dark, *i.e.*,
Reduced Visual Acuity

Many AIDS patients are commonly seen with damage of the eyes. The main pathoconditions manifesting in the region of the eyes are cotton-wool leukopathia, cytomegalovirus retinitis, retinal periphlebitis, toxoplasmic retinitis, and chorio-retinitis. In the initial stage of AIDS, there are usually no optic symptoms. However, cotton-wool leukopathia may present in the early prodromal stage accompanying fever. The later stages of this disease may be accompanied by retinal necrosis, hemorrhage, and atrophy. The manifestations are gradual loss of sight, dimming and blurring of vision, and even blindness.

A. Disease Causes, Disease Mechanisms

The causes of this disease are mostly deficiency and vacuity of the viscera and bowels, qi and blood and external attack by toxic evils. This results in phlegm turbidity and toxic evils accumulating internally. If turbid qi attacks the clear portals (*i.e.*, the sense organs and in this case more specifically the eyes), this may cause fogging of vision or blindness. If qi and blood are deficient and vacuous, they may not be able to promote blood circulation. This results in qi stagnation and blood stasis and obstruction and stagnation in the eye network vessels. If there is deficiency and vacuity of the liver and kidneys, essence and blood may be deficient and consumed. Likewise, if heart and spleen are both vacuous, qi and blood may be insufficient. Thus the eyes lack nourishment. All these may lead to the occurrence of this disease.

B. Differentiation & Treatment

1. *Zuo Xie Shang Fan*
Turbid Evils Attack Upward

Clinical manifestations: Vision dim and dark or shifting dark spots in front of the eyes, examination shows inflammatory exudation, oppression and fullness of the chest and epigastrium, poor appetite, yellow urine, a yellow slimy tongue fur, and a soggy, rapid pulse

Treatment principles: Clear heat and eliminate dampness, transform turbidity and brighten the eyes

Guiding formula: *San Ren Tang Jia Jian*

Medicinals: Talcum (*Hua Shi*), Semen Coicis Lachryma-jobi (*Sheng Yi Ren*), Semen Pruni Armeniacae (*Xing Ren*), Medulla Tetrapanacis Papyriferi (*Tong Cao*), Fructus Amomi Cardamomi (*Bai Kou Ren*), Herba Lophatheri Gracilis (*Zhu Ye*), Cortex Magnoliae Officinalis (*Hou Po*), Rhizoma Pinelliae Ternatae (*Ban Xia*), Scapus Eriocaulonis Buergeriani (*Gu Jing Cao*), Semen Astragali Complanati (*Sha Yuan Zi*)

Formula explanation: Talcum disinhibits dampness and clears heat. Semen Coicis Lachryma-jobi blandly seeps, fortifies the spleen, and disinhibits dampness. Semen Pruni Armeniacae, bitter and acrid, lightly opens the upper burner. If qi is transformed, dampness will also be transformed. Medulla Tetrapanacis Papyriferi and Herba Lophatheri Gracilis clear heat, disinhibit dampness, and guide heat down and out. Fructus Amomi Cardamomi moves the qi and transforms dampness. Cortex Magnoliae Officinalis and Rhizoma Pinelliae Ternatae move the qi, dry dampness, and fortify the spleen. Adding Scapus Eriocaulonis Buergeriani clears heat and brightens the eyes. And Semen Astragali Complanati enriches the liver and brightens the eyes.

Selected acupuncture/moxibustion points: *Jing Ming* (Bl 1)⊥, *Qui Hou* (M-HN-8)⊥, *Zu San Li* (St 36)⊥, *Yin Ling Quan* (Sp 9)⊥, & *He Gu* (LI 4)⊥

Formula rationale: Draining *Jing Ming* is chosen to course and free the channels and network vessels and brightens the eyes. *Qiu Hou* is an extra-channel point. It effectively treats eye diseases and brightens the eyes. Draining *Zu San Li* clears heat, eliminates evils, and scatters nodulation. *Yin Ling Quan* disinhibits dampness, fortifies the spleen, and transforms turbidity. Draining *He Gu* clears heat and resolves evil toxins. Used together, these points clear heat and expel dampness, transform turbidity and brighten the eyes.

2. *Qi Zhi Xue Yu*
Qi Stagnation, Blood Stasis

Clinical manifestations: Dark spots moving in front of the eyes, blurring of vision with gradual diminishment of sight, eye examination shows exudation, edema, and hemorrhage, chest andlateral costal distention and pain, dizziness, a bitter taste in the mouth and dry throat, static spots on the sides of the tongue, and a bound or choppy pulse

Treatment principles: Clear heat and course the liver, transform stasis and brighten the eyes

Guiding formula: *Xue Fu Zhu Yu Tang Jia Jian*

Medicinals: Semen Pruni Persicae (*Tao Ren*), Flos Carthami Tinctorii (*Hong Hua*), Radix Angelicae Sinensis (*Dang Gui*), uncooked Radix Rehmanniae (*Sheng Di*), Radix Ligustici Wallichii (*Chuan Xiong*), Radix Rubrus Paeoniae Lactiflorae (*Chi Shao*), Radix Achryranthis Bidentatae (*Niu Xi*), Radix Platycodi Grandiflori (*Jie Geng*), Radix Bupleuri (*Chai Hu*), Flos Buddleiae Officinalis (*Mi Meng Hua*), Radix Glycyrrhizae (*Gan Cao*)

Formula explanation: In this formula, Semen Pruni Persicae, Flos Carthami Tinctorii, and Radix Ligustici Wallichii quicken the blood and transform stasis. Uncooked Radix Rehmanniae clears heat, nourishes yin, engenders fluids, and stops thirst. Radix Rubrus Paeoniae Lactiflorae clears heat, resolves toxins, and transforms stasis. Radix Achyranthis Bidentatae guides the blood, moves it downward, and transforms stasis. Radix Platycodi Grandiflori and Radix Bupleuri course the liver, loosen the chest, and move the qi. Adding Flos Buddleiae Officinalis clears the liver and brightens the eyes. And Radix Glycyrrhizae regulates and harmonizes the preceding medicinals.

Selected acupuncture/moxibustion points: *Jing Ming* (Bl 1)⊥, *Zan Zhu* (Bl 2)⊥, *Ge Shu* (Bl 17)⊥, *Xue Hai* (Sp 10)⊥, & *Shan Zhong* (CV 17)⊥

Formula rationale: Draining *Jing Ming* recedes opacity and scatters stasis, relaxes the sinews and quickens the network vessels. Draining *Zan Zhu* frees the *luo* and brightens the eyes. Draining *Ge Shu* and *Xue Hai* quickens the blood and scatters stasis. *Shan Zhong* loosens the chest and rectifies the qi. Used together, these points have the ability to rectify the qi, transform phlegm, and brighten the eyes.

3. *Gan Shen Kui Xu*
Liver/Kidney Deficiency & Vacuity

Clinical manifestations: Dim and dark vision, dark spots in front of the eyes, flowers dancing in the air, inside the eyes dry and grating or even blindness, eye examination may show changes in the retina or choroid including atrophy, dizziness, tinnitus, night blindness, profuse dreaming, low back and knee soreness and weakness, a red tongue with thin fur, and a fine pulse

Treatment principles: Supplement and boost the liver and kidneys, boost the essence and brighten the eyes

Guiding formula: *Qi Ju Di Huang Wan Jia Jian*

Medicinals: Fructus Lycii Chinensis (*Gou Qi Zi*), Flos Chrysanthemi (*Ju Hua*), prepared Radix Rehmanniae (*Shu Di*), Fructus Corni Officinalis (*Shan Zhu Yu*), Rhizoma Alismatis (*Ze Xie*), Cortex Radicis Moutan (*Dan Pi*), Ramulus Loranthi Seu Visci (*Sang Shen*), Fructus Schizandrae Chinensis (*Wu Wei Zi*), Radix Angelicae Sinensis (*Dang Gui*)

Formula explanation: Fructus Lycii Chinensis and Flos Chrysanthemi nourish the liver and brighten the eyes. Prepared Radix Rehmanniae enriches and supplements kidney yin. Fructus Corni Officinalis nourishes the liver and kidneys and boosts the essence. Cortex Radicis Moutan and Rhizoma Alismatis clear and discharge vacuous fire from the liver and kidneys. Radix Angelicae Sinensis nourishes and quickens the blood. Ramulus Loranthi Seu Visci enriches yin and brightens the eyes by nourishing the liver. Fructus Schizandrae Chinensis enriches liver and kidney yin. Used together, these medicinals supplement and boost liver and kidney yin and brighten the eyes.

Selected acupuncture/moxibustion points: *Jing Ming* (Bl 1)т, *Tong Zi Liao* (GB 1)т, *Guang Ming* (GB 37)т, *Gan Shu* (Bl 18)т, & *Shen Shu* (Bl 23)т

Formula rationale: *Jing Ming* and *Tong Zi Liao* are main points for treating eye diseases. They clear the liver and brighten the eyes. *Guang Ming* is the network point of the foot *shao yang* channel. Supplementing it frees the network and brightens the eyes. *Gan Shu* and *Shen Shu*

supplement and boost the liver and kidneys, enrich yin and brighten the eyes.

4. *Xin Pi Liang Xu*
Heart/Spleen Dual Vacuity

Clinical manifestations: Eye symptoms the same as before, dizziness, poor appetite, lassitude of the spirit, lack of strength, shortness of breath, heart palpitations, loss of sleep, a lustreless facial complexion, a pale tongue with thin fur, and a fine, weak pulse

Treatment principles: Supplement and boost the heart and spleen, nourish the blood and brighten the eyes

Guiding formula: *Ren Shen Yang Ying Tang Jia Jian*

Medicinals: Radix Codonopsis Pilosulae (*Dang Shen*), Rhizoma Atractylodis Macrocephalae (*Bai Zhu*), Sclerotium Poriae Cocos (*Fu Ling*), Radix Angelicae Sinensis (*Dang Gui*), prepared Radix Rehmanniae (*Shu Di*), Radix Albus Paeoniae Lactiflorae (*Bai Shao*), Radix Ligustici Wallichii (*Chuan Xiong*), Fructus Schizandrae Chinensis (*Wu Wei Zi*), Radix Polygalae Tenuifoliae (*Yuan Zhi*), Placenta Hominis (*Zi He Che*), Gelatinum Cornu Cervi (*Lu Jiao Jiao*), Radix Salviae Miltiorrhizae (*Dan Shen*), Radix Glycyrrhizae (*Gan Cao*)

Formula explanation: In this formula, *Si Jun Zi Tang* fortifies the spleen and boosts the qi. *Si Wu Tang* supplements and regulates the blood and nourishes the heart. Fructus Schizandrae Chinensis and Radix Polygalae Tenuifoliae guard the heart and quiet the spirit. Placenta Hominis and Gelatinum Cornu Cervi supplement the essence, boost the qi, and nourish the blood with flesh and blood from living sources. Radix Salviae Miltiorrhizae quickens and nourishes the blood. And Radix Glycyrrhizae harmonizes the center. Used together, these medicinals have the ability to boost the qi and engender blood, nourish the blood and brighten the eyes.

Selected acupuncture/moxibustion points: *Jing Ming* (Bl 1)т, *Cheng Qi* (St 1)т, *Xin Shu* (Bl 15)т, *Shen Men* (Ht 7)т, & *Zu San Li* (St 36)т

Formula rationale: *Jing Ming* used in combination with *Cheng Qi* frees the flow of the channels and quickens the network vessels, clears the liver and brightens the eyes. Supplementing *Xin Shu* nourishes heart blood. *Zu San Li* supplements the spleen and stomach, transforms and engenders qi and blood. *Shen Men* is the *yuan* source point of the heart channel. Supplementing it nourishes heart blood and tranquilizes heart spirit. Used together, these points supplement and boost the heart and spleen, nourish the blood and brighten the eyes.

XVI. *Ji Ju*
Accumulations & Gatherings, *i.e.*, Abdominal Masses

In the full blown AIDS stage, patients's liver and spleen are typically affected and hence are swollen and enlarged. This is mainly the result of secondary infections and tumors of the liver and spleen. Many AIDS patients (also) have a previous history of hepatitis. In addition, mycobacterial, cryptococcal, and cytomegalovirus infections very commonly affect the liver and spleen causing chronic active hepatitis, cirrhosis, and Kaposi's sarcoma of the these two organs. Laboratory tests show rises in transaminase and alkaline phosphatase (AKP).

A. Disease Causes, Disease Mechanisms

This disease is usually caused by the invasion of pestilential toxic evils and deficiency and vacuity of righteous qi. If evils stagnate chronically and are not expelled, this will result in deficiency and vacuity of the viscera and bowels, qi and blood, their functions becoming imregulated. If the qi mechanism becomes obstructed and stagnant, blood stasis will arise internally or be accompanied by phlegm turbidity. The vessels and network vessels become stuffed and jammed. If phlegm turbidity and qi and blood mutually wrestle and knot for a prolonged time, this will give rise to accumulations and gatherings.

B. Differentiation & Treatment

1. *Qi Zhi Xue Yu*
Qi Stagnation, Blood Stasis

Clinical manifestations: Masses inside the abdomen, soft and not hard, fixed and not movable, or distention and pain, emaciation, lack of strength, a dark tongue or static spots with a thin, white fur, and a fine, choppy pulse

Treatment principles: Rectify the qi and quicken the blood, disperse accumulation and scatter nodulation

Guiding formula: *Ge Xia Zhu Yu Tang Jia Jian*

Medicinals: Radix Angelicae Sinensis (*Dang Gui*), Radix Ligustici Wallichii (*Chuan Xiong*), Semen Pruni Persicae (*Tao Ren*), Flos Carthami Tinctorii (*Hong Hua*), Rhizoma Corydalis Yanhusuo (*Yan Hu Suo*), Radix Auklandiae (*Mu Xiang*), Radix Linderae Strychnifoliae (*Wu Yao*), Sclerotium Poriae Cocos (*Fu Ling*), Rhizoma Cyperi Rotundi (*Xiang Fu*), Rhizoma Sparganii (*San Leng*), Rhizoma Curcumae Zedoariae (*E Zhu*), Radix Glycyrrhizae (*Gan Cao*)

Formula explanation: In this formula, Radix Angelicae Sinensis and Radix Ligustici Wallichii quicken the blood and transform stasis. Semen Pruni Persicae and Flos Carthami Tinctorii crack the blood and eliminate stasis. Rhizoma Cyperi Rotundi, Radix Linderae Strychnifoliae, Radix Auklandiae, and Rhizoma Corydalis Yanhusuo course the liver, rectify the qi, and stop pain. This is aided by Sclerotium Poriae Cocos which boosts the qi and fortifies the spleen. Radix Glycyrrhizae rectifys and harmonizes the preceding medicinals. Adding Rhizoma Sparganii and Rhizoma Curcumae Zedoariae quickens the blood, transforms stasis, disperses masses, and transforms accumulations.

Selected acupuncture/moxibustion points: *Shan Zhong* (CV 17)⊥, *Qi Hai* (CV 6)⊥, *Zhang Men* (Liv 13)⊥, *Xue Hai* (Sp 10)⊥, & *Ge Shu* (Bl 17)⊥

Formula rationale: *Shan Zhong* is chosen to course the liver, rectify the qi, and loosen the chest. Draining *Qi Hai* rectifies the qi and scatters nodulation. Draining *Xue Hai* quickens the blood and transforms stasis. Draining *Zhang Men* courses the liver and rectifys the spleen. And draining *Ge Shu* quickens the blood, transforms stasis, and frees the network vessels.

2. *Zheng Xu Yu Jie*
Righteous Vacuous, Stasis & Nodulation

Clinical manifestations: Hard masses with severe aching and pain which worsen gradually, a sallow yellow or dark facial complexion, bodily emaciation, exhausted, weary, lack of strength, a dark purple tongue with thin or no fur, and a deep, fine pulse

Treatment principles: Supplement and boost qi and blood, transform stasis and disperse accumulation

Guiding formula: *Ba Zhen Tang* plus *Hua Ji Wan Jia Jian*

Medicinals: Radix Codonopsis Pilosulae (*Dang Shen*), Rhizoma Atractylodis Macrocephalae (*Bai Zhu*), Sclerotium Poriae Cocos (*Fu Ling*), Radix Angelicae Sinensis (*Dang Gui*), Radix Ligustici Wallichii (*Chuan Xiong*), Radix Albus Paeoniae Lactiflorae (*Bai Shao*), prepared Radix Rehmanniae (*Shu Di*), Rhizoma Sparganii (*San Leng*), Rhizoma Curcumae Zedoariae (*E Zhu*), Rhizoma Cyperi Rotundi (*Xiang Fu*), Feces Trogopterori Seu Pteromi (*Wu Ling Zhi*), Semen Arecae Catechu (*Bing Lang*), Radix Glycyrrhizae (*Gan Cao*)

Formula explanation: In this formula, *Si Jun Zi Tang* supplements the center, boosts the qi, and fortifies the spleen. *Si Wu Tang* supplements the blood and nourishes the liver, regulates the blood and moves stasis. Rhizoma Sparganii and Rhizoma Curcumae Zedoariae transform stasis and disperse accumulation. Rhizoma Cyperi Rotundi and Semen Arecae Catechu course the liver, rectify the qi, and scatter nodulation. Feces Trogopterori Seu Pteromi quickens the blood and eliminates stasis in order to stop pain. When the above medicinals are used together, they support the righteous and supplement vacuity, transform stasis and disperse accumulations.

Selected acupuncture/moxibustion points: *Gan Shu* (Bl 18)⊤, *Pi Shu* (Bl 20)⊤, *Ge Shu* (Bl 17)⊥, *Xue Hai* (Sp 10)⊥, *Zhang Men* (Liv 13)⊥, & *Yin Ling Quan* (Sp 9)⊤

Formula rationale: Supplementing *Gan Shu* nourishes the blood. Supplementing *Pi Shu* supplements the center and boosts the qi. *Yin Ling Quan* is the sea point of the spleen channel. It is able to fortify the spleen and supplement the blood. Draining *Ge Shu* quickens the blood and transforms stasis. Draining *Xue Hai* moves and quickens the blood and stops pain. Draining *Zhang Men* courses the liver and rectifys the spleen, eliminates stasis and transforms accumulations.

XVII. *Lin Zheng*
Stranguria

Difficult urination is also one of the main symptoms in the later stages of AIDS. It is usually caused by chronic problems of the kidneys and bladder. The former (*i.e.*, problems of the kidneys) are usually the result of recurrent opportunistic infections (in turn) caused by *Monilia albicans, Cryptococcus, Aspergillus, Moniliformis* and Cytomegalovirus and Kaposi's sarcoma. Examination may reveal abnormal glomeruli and basement membrane deposits. Likewise, patients typically have proteinuria and eventually renal failure. The latter (*i.e.*, problems of the bladder) comprise infections of the urinary system, most often cystitis and urethritis.

A. Disease Causes, Disease Mechanisms

This disease is usually caused by pestilential evils internally hidden for a long time which give rise internally to damp heat which pours down to the bladder. Qi transformation loses its management and the water passageways are inhibited. Or in chronic cases, dual deficiency of the spleen and kidneys results in qi transformation being inhibited. This results in urination being frequent, short, and astringent. There is dribbling, dripping, and pricking pain. Thus the occurrence of this disease.

B. Differentiation & Treatment

1. *Xia Jiao Shi Re*
Lower Burner Damp Heat

Clinical manifestations: Urination burning hot, short, scant urine, frequent urination, urinary urgency, urinary pain, a bitter mouth, low back pain, defecation not smooth, a red tongue with a yellow, slimy fur, and a soggy, rapid pulse

Treatment principles: Clear heat and disinhibit dampness, free and disinhibit urination

Guiding formula: *Ba Zheng San Jia Jian*

Medicinals: Caulis Akebiae (*Mu Tong*), Semen Plantaginis (*Che Qian Zi*), Talcum (*Hua Shi*), Herba Polygoni Aviculari (*Bian Xu*), Herba Dianthi (*Qu Mai*), Rhizoma Imperatae Cyclindricae (*Bai Mao Geng*), Fructus Gardeniae Jasminoidis (*Shan Zhi*), Radix Et Rhizoma Rhei (*Da Huang*), Radix Glycyrrhizae (*Gan Cao*)

Formula explanation: In this formula, Fructus Gardeniae Jasminoidis and Semen Plantaginis clear heat, resolve toxins, and disinhibit dampness. Herba Polygoni Aviculari and Herba Dianthi clear heat and disinhibit dampness, disinhibit water and free *lin* or stranguria. Adding Radix Et Rhizoma Rhei frees the bowels and drains heat, leads damp heat out via urination. Talcum is used to clear heat and disinhibit dampness to strengthen the disinhibition of water. Rhizoma Imperatae Cyclindricae clears heat and cools the blood. And Radix Glycyrrhizae harmonizes the middle, resolves toxins, and also prevents the above bitter, cold (medicinals) from damaging the stomach.

Selected acupuncture/moxibustion points: *Pang Guang Shu* (Bl 28)⊥, *Zhong Ji* (CV 3)⊥, *Yin Ling Quan* (Sp 9)⊥, *Xing Jian* (Liv 2)⊥, & *San Yin Jiao* (Sp 6)⊥

Formula rationale: Draining *Pang Guang Shu* clears and disinhibits damp heat in the bladder. Draining *Zhong Ji* frees and disinhibits urination. Draining *Yin Ling Quan* fortifies the spleen and disinhibits dampness. Draining *Xing Jian* courses the liver and clears heat. And draining *San Yin Jiao* clears and disinhibits damp turbidity in the lower burner.

2. *Zheng Xu Xue Yu*
Righteous Vacuity, Blood Stasis

Clinical manifestations: Inhibited urination or even complete inability to void, lassitude of the spirit, lack of strength, extreme emaciation, a dark, pale tongue or static spots, and a deep, fine, choppy pulse

Treatment principles: Supplement the center and boost the qi, free and disinhibit the water passageways

Guiding formula: *Dai Di Dang Wan Jia Jian*

Medicinals: Radix Astragali Membranacei (*Huang Qi*), Radix Codonopsis Pilosulae (*Dang Shen*), Rhizoma Atractylodis

Macrocephalae (*Bai Zhu*), Radix Angelicae Sinensis (*Dang Gui*), Semen Plantaginis (*Che Qian Zi*), Radix Bupleuri (*Chai Hu*), Squama Manitis Pentadactylis (*Chuan Shan Jia*), Radix Et Rhizoma Rhei (*Da Huang*), Semen Pruni Persicae (*Tao Ren*), Cortex Cinnamomi (*Rou Gui*), Radix Achyrantis Bidentatae (*Niu Xi*)

Formula explanation: In this formula, Radix Astragali Membranacei and Radix Codonopsis Pilosulae boost the qi and supplement the middle to aid qi transformation. Rhizoma Atractylodis Macrocephalae fortifies the spleen and disinhibits dampness. Radix Angelicae Sinensis supplements and quickens the blood. Radix Bupleuri courses and disinhibits the qi mechanism. Semen Plantaginis and Radix Achyranthis Bidentatae transform dampness and disinhibit water, free and disinhibit urination. Squama Manitis Pentadactylis, Radix Et Rhizoma Rhei, and Semen Pruni Persicae move stasis and scatter nodulation, free and disinhibit the water passageways. Adding a little Cortex Cinnamomi warms and supplements the lower source to inspire and enhearten kidney qi. These medicinals together both attack and supplement at the same time, thus freeing and disinhibiting urination.

Selected acupuncture/moxibustion points: *Pang Guang Shu* (Bl 28)⊥, *Zhong Ji* (CV 3)⊥, *Tai Xi* (Ki 3)⊤, *Qi Hai* (CV 6)⊤, & *Shui Dao* (St 28)⊥

Formula rationale: Draining *Pang Guang Shu* clears and disinhibits the bladder, transforms stasis and frees the network vessels. Draining *Zhong Ji* frees and disinhibits urination. Supplementing *Tai Xi* enriches and supplements kidney yin. Supplementing *Qi Hai* banks up and supplements righteous qi. And draining *Shui Dao* disinhibits water and frees stranguria.

XVIII. *Xin Ji*
Heart Palpitations

In the full blown AIDS stage, due to severe depression of immunologic function, patients may also have opportunistic infections of the heart. This may manifest as pericarditis, myocarditis, endocarditis, etc. Metastatic Kaposi's sarcoma within the heart may also affect the cardiac muscle, coronary arteries, and the pericardium. This is why patients frequently present heart symptoms such as palpitations, cardiac insufficiency, etc.

A. Disease Causes, Disease Mechanisms

This disease is often caused by deficiency and vacuity of the righteous qi and invasion of external evils. Evil toxins may accumulate internally and trouble the heart spirit above, thus causing heart palpitations. Or, if heart blood is insufficient, the heart may lose its nourishment and not be able to treasure or store the spirit. Or, if heart yang does not rise with force and spirit, it cannot warm and nourish the heart vessels. Or, if spleen and kidney yang are vacuous, they cannot warm and transform water dampness. In this case, fluids stop up and disturb above. Heart yang oppressed and troubled or heart yang not rising with force and spirit may lead to blood stasis obstructing the network vessels and hence to the arisal of heart palpitations.

B. Differentiation & Treatment

1. *Xin Xue Bu Zu*
Heart Blood Insufficiency

Clinical manifestations: Palpitations, dizziness, blurred vision, lustreless facial complexion, mind not rising up with force and spirit, lassitude of the spirit, lack of strength, a pale tongue, and a fine, weak pulse

Treatment principles: Supplement the blood and nourish the heart, quiet the spirit and stabilize palpitations

Guiding formula: *Zhi Gan Cao Tang Jia Jian*

Medicinals: mix-fried Radix Glycyrrhizae (*Zhi Gan Cao*), Radix Panacis Ginseng (*Ren Shen*), Ramulus Cinnamomi (*Gui Zhi*), Rhizoma Atractylodis Macrocephalae (*Bai Zhu*), Gelatinum Corii Asini (*E Jiao*), uncooked Rhizoma Zingiberis (*Sheng Jiang*), Semen Zizyphi Spinosae (*Suan Zao Ren*), Radix Polygalae Tenuifoliae (*Yuan Zhi*), prepared Radix Rehmanniae (*Di Huang*), Tuber Ophiopogonis Japonicae (*Mai Dong*), Fructus Zizyphi Jujubae (*Da Zao*)

Formula explanation: In this formula, mix-fried Radix Glycyrrhizae boosts the qi and nourishes the heart. Adding Radix Panacis Ginseng, Rhizoma Atractylodis Macrocephalae, and Fructus Zizyphi Jujubae supplements the qi and boosts the stomach to aid the source of qi and blood engenderment and transformation. Gelatinum Corii Asini, prepared Radix Rehmanniae, and Tuber Ophiopogonis Japonicae enrich and nourish yin blood to fill and nourish the blood vessels. Semen Zizyphi Spinosae and Radix Polygalae quiet the spirit and stabilize palpitation. Adding Ramulus Cinnamomi and uncooked Rhizoma Zingiberis warms yang, frees the vessels, and promotes vigorous blood circulation. Used together, these medicinals promote heart blood, fill sufficiency, and obtain the quiet of the heart spirit, thus automatically stopping heart palpitations.

Selected acupuncture/moxibustion points: *Xin Shu* (Bl 15)T, *Ge Shu* (Bl 17)T, *Tong Li* (Ht 5)T, *Shen Men* (Ht 7)T, & *Zu San Li* (St 36)T

Formula rationale: Supplementing *Xin Shu* is able to boost heart blood. Supplementing the meeting point of the blood, *Ge Shu*, is able to fill and nourish heart blood. *Tong Li* boosts heart qi and heart blood. *Shen Men* nourishes the heart and clams the spirit. *Zu San Li* strengthens the transportation of the spleen and stomach, transforms and engenders qi and blood.

2. *Xin Yang Bu Zhen*
Heart Yang Not Rising with Gusto

Clinical manifestations: Heart palpitations, chest oppression, shortness of breath, body cold, limbs chilled, lassitude of the spirit, lack of strength, a pale tongue, and an vacuous, weak pulse

Treatment principles: Warm and supplement heart yang, tranquilize the heart and quiet the spirit

Guiding formula: *Gui Zhi Gan Cao Long Gu Mu Li Tang*

Medicinals: Ramulus Cinnamomi (*Gui Zhi*), Os Draconis (*Long Gu*), Concha Ostreae (*Mu Li*), mix-fried Radix Glycyrrhizae (*Zhi Gan Cao*)

Formula explanation: In this formula, Ramulus Cinnamomi, acrid and warm, rises up heart yang with gusto, promotes the blood, and frees and courses the vessels. Mix-fried Radix Glycyrrhizae, sweet and warm, relaxes irritation and nourishes the heart. Assistance from Os Draconis and Concha Ostreae heavily settles the heart, quiets the spirit, and stabilizes the emotions.

For those whose condition is severe with continuous asthma, cold sweats dripping wet, and counterflow chilling of the four limbs, add Radix Panacis Ginseng (*Ren Shen*) and Radix Lateralis Praeparatus Aconiti Carmichaeli (*Fu Zi*) to return yang and secure desertion.

Selected acupuncture/moxibustion points: *Xin Shu* (Bl 15)▵, *Shen Men* (Ht 7)⊤, *Qi Hai* (CV 6)▵, & *He Gu* (LI 4)⊤

Formula rationale: Supplementing *Xin Shu* boosts heart blood. *Shen Men* is the source point of the heart channel. Supplementing it can nourish the heart and quiet the spirit. Moxaing *Qi Hai* banks and supplements simultaneously the body's source qi. And *He Gu* is chosen to free the channels and activate the network vessels, to promote and upbear heart yang.

For those with heart yang on the verge of desertion, moxa *Shen Que* (CV 8) and *Guan Yuan* (CV 4) to return yang and secure desertion. Also drain *Nei Guan* (Per 6) to strengthen the heart and quiet the spirit.

3. *Shui Qi Ling Xin*
Water Qi Insulting the Heart

Clinical manifestations: Heart palpitations, asthma, chest and lateral costal oppression and fullness, lower limb edema, body cold, limbs chilled, short, scant urine, white, slimy tongue fur, and a wiry, slippery pulse

Treatment principles: Warm and free heart yang, transform qi and move water

Guiding formula: *Zhen Wu Tang Jia Wei*

Medicinals: Radix Lateralis Praeparatus Aconiti Carmichaeli (*Fu Zi*), Sclerotium Poriae Cocos (*Fu Ling*), Rhizoma Atractylodis Macrocephalae (*Bai Zhu*), Ramulus Cinnamomi (*Gui Zhi*), mix-fried Radix Glycyrrhizae (*Zhi Can Cao*), Radix Albus Paeoniae Lactiflorae (*Bai Shao*), uncooked Rhizoma Zingiberis (*Sheng Jiang*)

Formula explanation: In this formula, Radix Lateralis Praeparatus Aconiti Carmichaeli, very acrid, very hot, warms yang, transforms qi, and moves water. It is assisted by Ramulus Cinnamomi which warms and frees heart yang. Uncooked Rhizoma Zingiberis, acrid and warm, aids Radix Lateralis Praeparatus Aconiti Carmichaeli in warming yang and transforming qi. Rhizoma Atractylodis Macrocephalae boosts the qi, fortifies the spleen, and disinhibits water. Radix Albus Paeoniae Lactiflorae nourishes yin and disinhibits water, lightly harmonizes Radix Lateralis Praeparatus Aconiti Carmichaeli's acrid dryness. Mix-fried Radix Glycyrrhizae boosts the qi and nourishes the heart as well as rectifys and harmonizes the preceding medicinals.

Selected acupuncture/moxibustion points: *Xin Shu* (Bl 15)т, *Shen Men* (Ht 7)т, *Yin Ling Quan* (Sp 9)⊥, *Guan Yuan* (CV 4)▵, & *Shui Fen* (CV 9)▵

Formula rationale: Supplementing *Xin Shu* boosts heart qi. *Shen Men* tranquilizes the heart and quiets the spirit. Draining *Yin Ling Quan* fortifies the spleen, transforms dampness, and disinhibits water. Moxaing *Guan Yuan* is able to bank and supplement the source qi, warm yang and transform dampness. Moxaing *Shui Fen* moves the qi and disinhibits water.

4. *Xin Xue Yu Zu*
Heart Blood Stasis & Obstruction

Clinical manifestations: Heart palpitations, shortness of breath, stuffy chest and pain, or purplish lips and nails, a dark tongue or static spots, and a choppy or bound or regularly intermittent pulse

Treatment principles: Quicken the blood and transform stasis, stop pain and stabilize palpitation

Guiding formula: *Tao Ren Hong Hua Jian Jia Jian*

Medicinals: Semen Pruni Persicae (*Tao Ren*), Flos Carthami Tinctorii (*Hong Hua*), Radix Salviae Miltiorrhizae (*Dan Shen*), Radix Rubrus Paeoniae Lactiflorae (*Chi Shao*), Radix Ligustici Wallichii (*Chuan Xiong*), Rhizoma Corydalis Yanhusuo (*Yan Hu Suo*), prepared Radix Rehmanniae (*Shu Di*), Radix Angelicae Sinensis (*Dang Gui*)

Formula explanation: In this formula, Semen Pruni Persicae, Flos Carthami Tinctorii, and Radix Rubrus Paeoniae Lactiflorae quicken the blood and transform stasis. Radix Angelicae Sinensis nourishes and quickens the blood. Radix Salviae Miltiorrhizae quickens the blood and frees the vessels. Rhizoma Corydalis Yanhusuo and prepared Radix Rehmanniae enrich yin and nourish the heart. Used together, these

185

medicinals categorically transform stasis, stop pain, and stabilize palpitation.

For those with deficiency and vacuity of both qi and blood, add Radix Astragali Membranacei (*Huang Qi*), Radix Codonopsis Pilosulae (*Dang Shen*), Rhizoma Polygonati (*Huang Jing*), and Fructus Lycii Chinensis (*Gou Qi Zi*) to boost the qi and nourish the blood.

Selected acupuncture/moxibustion points: *Xin Shu* (Bl 15)⊤, *Shao Hai* (Ht 3)⊥, *Nei Guan* (Per 6)⊥, *He Gu* (LI 4)|, & *Xue Hai* (Sp 10)⊥

Formula rationale: Supplementing *Xin Shu* boosts the qi, quickens the blood, and transforms stasis. Draining *Shao Hai* frees the network vessels and stops pain. Draining *Nei Guan* eliminates stasis and frees the network vessels, tranquilizes the heart and quiets the spirit. And even supplementation and drainage of *He Gu* rectifys and supplements qi and blood.

XIX. *Chi Dai*
Dementia

In the later stages of AIDS, there is usually damage to the nervous system. Patients commonly present with the force of their concentration divided and scattered, memory impeded, loss of regulation, and even dementia. Nervous system complications due to AIDS are mainly localized in the brain, spinal chord, or peripheral nervous system. Opportunistic infections may cause cerebritis, meningitis, or myelitis. If there is lymph node swelling and enlargement and even tumors, this may lead to increase of intracranial pressure. In addition, malnutrition and disturbed metabolism can also cause nervous system disease. The causes of these infections are usually *Toxoplasma*, Cytomegalovirus, Herpes simplex virus, retrovirus, *Mycobacteria avium*, and *Cryptococcus neoformans*.

A. Disease Causes, Disease Mechanisms

The causes of this disease in chronic cases is mostly due to viscera and bowel, qi and blood deficiency and vacuity, the accumulation of dampness transforming into phlegm, and phlegm turbidity arising internally. Or, liver depression combined with spleen/stomach deficiency and vacuity may result in phlegm dampness stuffing and obstruction. This disturbs the clear portals above, eventually leading to dementia. Further, in the final stage of AIDS, due to deficiency and consumption of source qi, qi and blood are insufficient to moisten and nourish heart spirit. The brain marrow is not filled and this results in the manifestation of this pathocondition.

B. Differentiation & Treatment

1. *Tan Shi Zu Qiao*
Phlegm Dampness Obstructing the Portals

Clinical manifestations: Stupid and dull-witted like a fool or emotional depression accompanied by insomnia, a heavy sensation in the head, dizziness, copious phlegm or even unconsciousness, a pale tongue with thick, slimy fur, and a slippery, weak or wiry, slippery pulse

Treatment principles: Rectify the qi and resolve depression, wash away phlegm and open the portals

Guiding formula: *Zhuan Dai Dan Jia Jian*

Medicinals: Radix Panacis Ginseng (*Ren Shen*), Radix Angelicae Sinensis (*Dang Gui*), Rhizoma Cyperi Rotundi (*Xiang Fu*), Rhizoma Pinelliae Ternatae (*Ban Xia*), Rhizoma Arisaematis (*Nan Xing*), Semen Zizyphi Spinosae (*Suan Zao Ren*), Rhizoma Acori Graminei (*Shi Chang Pu*), Sclerotium Pararadicis Poriae Cocos (*Fu Shen*), Radix Bupleuri (*Chai Hu*), Semen Biotae Orientalis (*Bai Zi Ren*)

Formula explanation: In this formula, Radix Panacis Ginseng supplements the middle and boosts the qi. Radix Bupleuri and Rhizoma Cyperi Rotundi course the liver and rectify the qi, resolve depression and diffuse the portals. Rhizoma Pinelliae Ternatae and Rhizoma Arisaematis clear the heart and wash away phlegm to expel turbid evils. Radix Angelicae Sinensis nourishes the blood. Semen Zizyphi Spinosae, Sclerotium Pararadicis Poriae Cocos, and Semen Biotae Orientalis tranquilize the heart and quiet the spirit. And Rhizoma Acori Graminei is chosen to transform phlegm and open the portals. Used together, these medicinals categorically wash away phlegm and open the portals, resolve depression and wake the spirit, and supplement and drain at the same time.

For those with phlegm turbidity obstructing the *luo* manifesting as epilepsy, one way is to use *Ding Xian Wan* to wash away phlegm and extinguish wind, open the portals and stabilize epilepsy.

Medicinals: Bile-processed Rhizoma Arisaematis (*Dan Nan Xing*), Rhizoma Pinelliae Ternatae (*Ban Xia*), Rhizoma Acori Graminei (*Shi Chang Pu*), Succus Bambusae (*Zhu Li*), Sclerotium Poriae Cocos (*Fu Ling*), Cinnabaris (*Chen Sha*), Succinum (*Hu Po*), Lumbricus (*Di Long*), Rhizoma Gastrodiae Elatae (*Tian Ma*), Buthus Martensis (*Quan Xie*), Bombyx Batryticatus (*Jiang Can*)

Formula explanation: Bile-processed Rhizoma Arisaematis, Rhizoma Pinelliae Ternatae, and Succus Bambusae break up phlegm and open the portals. Rhizoma Acori Graminei invigorates and upbears clear yang, arouses the spirit and washes away phlegm. Sclerotium Poriae Cocos fortifies the spleen and transforms dampness. Cinnabaris and Succinum heavily settle the heart and quiet the spirit. Rhizoma Gastrodiae Elatae, Buthus Martensi, and Bombyx Batryticatus level the liver, extinguish wind, and stop spasm.

Selected acupuncture/moxibustion points: *Shen Men* (Ht 7)|, *Da Ling* (Per 7)⊥, *Shan Zhong* (CV 17)⊥, *Feng Long* (St 40)⊥, *San Yin Jiao* (Sp 6)⊥, & *Yin Tang* (M-HN-3)⊥

Formula rationale: Even supplementation and drainage of *Shen Men* tranquilizes the heart and quiets the spirit. Draining *Da Ling* opens the portals and arouses the spirit. Draining *Shan Zhong* rectifies the qi and resolves depression. *Feng Long* downbears turbidity and transforms phlegm. *San Yin Jiao* fortifies the spleen and disinhibits dampness, eliminates phlegm and transforms turbidity. *Yin Tang* is an extra-channel point. Needling it using draining method arouses the brain and opens the portals.

For those accompanied by epilepsy, drain *Da Zhui* (GV 14) to wake the brain and clear the spirit, invigorate and upbear yang qi. Also drain the blood vessel at *Jiu Wei* (CV 15) to resolve depression and transform phlegm. Drain *Chang Qiang* (CV 1) to free the *luo* and stop spasm. For those attacked in the daytime, add *Shen Mai* (Bl 62). For those attacked at night, add *Zhao Hai* (Ki 6). Both points are meeting points of the eight vessels. Draining them is able to free and smooth the *qiao mai* and stop spasm.

2. *Xin Pi Liang Xu*
Heart/Spleen Dual Vacuity

Clinical manifestations: Dull like a fool, mind in a trance, injured by sadness, on verge of crying, chest oppression, vacuous vexation, insomnia, lassitude of the spirit, lack of strength, poor appetite, a pale tongue, and a deep, forceless pulse

Treatment principles: Fortify the spleen and nourish the heart, boost the qi and quiet the spirit

Guiding formula: *Yang Xin Tang* plus *Gan Mai Da Zao Tang Jia Jian*

Medicinals: Radix Panacis Ginseng (*Ren Shen*), Radix Dioscoreae Oppositae (*Shan Yao*), Sclerotium Pararadicis Poriae Cocos (*Fu Shen*), Radix Angelicae Sinensis (*Dang Gui*), Radix Albus Paeoniae Lactiflorae (*Bai Shao*), Semen Nelumbinis Nuciferae (*Lian Zi*), Radix Polygalae Tenuifoliae (*Yuan Zhi*), Semen Zizyphi Spinosae (*Suan Zao Ren*),

Fructus Levis Tritici Aestivi (*Fu Xiao Mai*), Fructus Zizyphi Jujubae (*Da Zao*), mix-fried Radix Glycyrrhizae (*Zhi Gan Cao*)

Formula explanation: In this formula, Radix Panacis Ginseng boosts the qi and fortifies the spleen, nourishes the heart and quiets the spirit. It is combined with Radix Dioscoreae Oppositae which assists the promotion of the spleen. Radix Albus Paeoniae Lactiflorae and Radix Angelicae Sinensis supplement the blood and nourish the heart. Sclerotium Pararadicis Poriae Cocos, Semen Nelumbinis Nuciferae, Radix Polygalae Tenuifoliae, and Semen Zizyphi Spinosae tranquilize the heart and quiet the spirit. Fructus Levis Tritici, sweet and neutral, relaxes irritation and nourishes the heart. Radix Glycyrrhizae and Fructus Zizyphi Jujubae supplement the center and boost the qi, rectify and harmonize the preceding medicinals.

Selected acupuncture/moxibustion points: *Xin Shu* (Bl 15)⊤, *Shen Men* (Ht 7)|, *Zu San Li* (St 36)⊤, *San Yin Jiao* (Sp 6)⊤, & *Bai Hui* (GV 20)⊤

Formula rationale: Supplementing *Xin Shu* can nourish the heart and tranquilize the spirit. *Shen Men* is the source point of the heart channel. Even supplementation and drainage of it is able to clear the heart and quiet the spirit. Supplementing *Zu San Li* fortifies the spleen and boosts the stomach, transforms and engenders the origin of qi and blood. *San Yin Jiao* supplements and boosts the heart and spleen, enriches yin and nourishes blood. *Bai Hui* boosts the qi and ascends yang to aid qi and blood being offered up to the head and brain.

6

Fu Zhong Xi Yi Zhi Liao Ai Zi Bing

The Treatment of AIDS With Combined Chinese-Western Medicine

In Traditional Chinese Medicine, the treatment of AIDS is still in its early period of clinical research. At present, it is still difficult to effect a radical cure. Because of serious immune deficiency, the occurrence of AIDS manifests injuries of every system and organ of the body, especially in the full blown AIDS stage. This easily results in various kinds of opportunistic infections and all kinds of malignant tumors. Further, patients' conditions worsen rapidly. Applying either only Chinese medicine or only Western medicine cannot control these various pathoconditions nor the underlying disease itself. Nor can it completely eradicate the pathogen (*i.e.*, HIV).

Therefore, in clinical practice, it is important to diagnose and treat with a combination of both traditional Chinese and modern Western medicines. Through a vast number of experiments, great progress has been made in showing the superiority of such a combination. Recently in China, rich experience has been accumulated in treating immune deficiencies and malignant tumors with this combination. These successes have led to the widespread idea of also curing AIDS with this combination.

For instance, in diagnosing AIDS, the 4 diagnoses or *si zhen* of TCM are not enough. Therefore, doctors can use Western diagnostic methods to aid in early and definite diagnosis. Also, Western medical tests can be used to verify the curative effect of various treatments, observe the immune function of the body, and monitor a treatment's antiviral activity. Thus one can evaluate the curative effect objectively and address the pathophysiological mechanisms of this disease.

Generally speaking, the combination of Western medicine and TCM is significantly effective in improving cure and survival rates. Available information indicates that Chinese medicine can relieve the toxicity and side effects of Western medicine. Also it can raise the survival rate by adjusting the function of the body systemically. The situation in foreign countries exemplifies this. Though Western doctors do not understand nor attempt to administer it, many AIDS patients in foreign countries independently seek acupuncture and other Chinese medical treatment. Because at present Western medicine has had no success in comprehensively treating AIDS, the relative advantages of Traditional Chinese Medicine have gained more and more attention in foreign countries. We believe it is necessary to use both modalities and apply them in combination. This has been proven effective. In this chapter, the combination of chemotherapy, radiation therapy and TCM is discussed. Also included in this chapter are proven, effective treatments for improving immunity.

I. *Zhong Yi Jie He Fang Zhi Hua Zhi*
Chinese Medicine Combined with Radiation & Chemotherapy

Presently, chemotherapy is a commonly applied therapy in the treatment of AIDS. However, because of its toxicity and lack of specificity, it can further injure the already deficient immunity of AIDS patients and inhibit the function of their bone marrow. This essential contradiction in therapy with chemotherapy is unavoidable. On the other hand, Chinese medicine can relieve these side effects by supplementing the righteous qi, strengthening disease resistance, and regulating the function of the body as a whole.

In China, the treatment of tumors with combined Chinese medicine and chemotherapy has recently made great headway. For example, great progress has been made in raising cure rates in the treatment of liver cancer with combined Chinese-Western medicine. Likewise, in full blown AIDS, many malignant tumors may arise. Therefore, radiation therapy is also commonly used to treat these. When TCM is combined with radiotherapy, it also can improve the amelioration rate, relieve radiation's toxicity, and enhance its effect by regulating function both locally and systemically.

Because of patients' systemic hypofunction, Traditional Chinese Medicine can be used to supplement the righteous qi and regulate the body's function before applying chemotherapy and radiation. Depending upon the individual situation, treatment with medicinals and acupuncture to improve immunity may be administered on the basis of a discrimination of patterns. In the course of treatment, Chinese medicine can reduce the side effects of radiation and chemotherapy. After chemotherapy and radiation, there may appear manifestations of empty yin or empty qi. The use of TCM can improve the systemic situation, the state of blood analysis, the function of individual organs, as well as relieve the patient's symptoms. Hence the treatment effect can be enhanced.

It is also worth mentioning that recent research has verified the fact that Chinese medicine can also strengthen the tumor-combatting effect of chemotherapy and radiation. At present, this fact has attracted the interest of researchers both in and outside of China. For instance, comprehensive application of herbal formulas and radiation has demonstrated a coordinated function in curing tumors. In the Hunan

Medical College Affiliated Hospital, injection of Radix Ligustici Wallichii (*Chuan Xiong*) and Flos Carthami Tinctorii (*Hong Hua*) was tested in the treatment of nasopharyngeal cancer. Results indicate that such injections strengthened the effect of radiation. Treated patients needed less radiation than those in the untreated control group. Moreover, the Medical Research Institute of the Chinese Academy of Science has reported that, when an extract of Sclerotium Poriae Cocos (*Fu Ling*) was administered with cyclophosphamide, inhibition of tumors was more effective than when cyclophosphamide was used alone.

At present, such research is only at its beginning stage. The mechanisms for how and why Chinese medicinals may enhance the function of chemotherapy and radiation are still not clear. Therefore, when applying Chinese medicinals with chemotherapy and radiation, the differentiation of patterns should be closely discriminated. In other words, based on pattern discrimination, Chinese medicine can be applied to strengthen the effect of chemotherapy and radiation and reduce their toxic and side effects. Hence their overall effect is enhanced.

II. *Ai Zi Bing Fang Zhi Hua Zhi Fu Zuo Yong De Zhi Liao*
The Treatment of the Side Effects of Radiation & Chemotherapy in AIDS

Radiation and chemotherapy are two commonly applied modern Western medical treatments. Since chemotherapeutic drugs are extremely toxic, especially inhibiting bone marrow, and since radiation is not specifically selective to its targets, these two treatment methods may further injure an already deficient immune system, thus presenting a contradiction in treatment. For instance, the present best drug for treating AIDS is AZT. But AZT can not only cause reactions in the gastrointestinal tract but also inhibit the bone marrow as well. This then results in severe bone marrow depression and anemia. To make matters worse, because AIDS patients' immune function is so low, the toxic effect of such chemotherapeutic agents may be all the more severe. Therefore, in clinical practice it is very appropriate to use Chinese herbal medicine and acupuncture/moxibustion in combination with these more modern therapies in order to protect the body and reduce the toxic or side effects.

According to TCM theory, chemotherapy and radiation's toxicity is categorized as hot toxic evils. These injure the essence and consume the qi, damage yin and scorch fluids. This may cause loss of regulation of the qi and blood, disharmony of the spleen and stomach, and injury and damage of the liver and kidneys. It may even inhibit the marrow, exhaust the brain, and obstruct and hinder the origin of qi and blood engenderment and transformation, thus resulting in various pathoconditions. Treatment should support the righteous and bank the root assisted by clearing heat and resolving toxins, cooling the blood and transforming stasis in order to categorically support the root and eliminate evil.

A. *Gu Sui Yi Zhi*
Bone Marrow Inhibition

1. *Qi Xue Xu Ruo*
Qi & Blood Vacuous & Weak

Clinical manifestations: Whole body exhausted and weary, dizziness, blurred vision, a somber white facial complexion, falling, faded hair, heart palpitations, a pale tongue with thin, white fur, and a fine, forceless pulse

Treatment principles: Boost the qi and nourish the blood, fortify the spleen and engender marrow

Guiding formula: *Ba Zhen Tang Jia Jian*

Medicinals: Radix Astragali Membranacei (*Huang Qi*), Radix

Codonopsis Pilosulae (*Dang Shen*), Sclerotium Poriae Cocos (*Fu Ling*), Rhizoma Atractylodis Macrocephlae (*Bai Zhu*), Radix Angelicae Sinensis (*Dang Gui*), Radix Albus Paeoniae Lactiflorae (*Bai Shao*), Caulis Milletiae Seu Spatholobi (*Ji Xue Teng*), Radix Rubiae Cordifoliae (*Qian Cao*), Fructus Psoraleae Corylifoliae (*Bu Gu Zhi*), Fructus Zizyphi Jujubae (*Da Zao*), mix-fried Radix Glycyrrhizae (*Zhi Gan Cao*)

Formula explanation: Radix Astragali Membranacei greatly supplements the source qi. Radix Codonopsis Pilosulae, sweet and warm, boosts the qi. Sclerotium Poriae Cocos and Rhizoma Atractylodis Macrocephalae fortify the spleen and dry dampness. Radix Angelicae Sinensis and Radix Albus Paeoniae Lactiflorae nourish the blood and harmonize the constructive. Fructus Zizyphi Jujubae regulates and harmonizes spleen and stomach qi. Mix-fried Radix Glycyrrhizae harmonizes the middle and boosts the qi. Adding Caulis Milletiae Seu Sptholobi and Radix Rubiae Cordifoliae nourishes and quickens the blood to engender marrow. And Fructus Psoraleae Corylifoliae supplements the kidneys and aids yang to produce hair. The entire formula together not only supplements both qi and blood but also fortifies the spleen and engenders marrow.

Selected acupuncture/moxibustion points: *Da Zhui* (GV 14)▵, *Zu San Li* (St 36)▵, *Xue Hai* (Sp 10)⊤, *He Gu* (LI 4)⊤, & *Ge Shu* (Bl 17)⊤

Formula rationale: Moxaing *Zu San Li* and *Da Zhui* can warm and supplement the qi and blood, bank the source and engender the marrow. *Xue Hai* can boost the spleen and conserve the blood, engender and nourish the blood. *He Gu* used with supplementation technique can boost the qi and ascend yang, move and engender the blood. And supplementing *Ge Shu* can nourish yin and blood and engender marrow.

2. *Gan Shen Yin Xu*
Liver/Kidney Yin Vacuity

Clinical manifestations: Dizziness, tinnitus, heart palpitations, disquietude, *i.e.*, restlessness, dry mouth with desire to drink, tidal fever, night sweats, or seminal emission, low back and knee soreness and weakness, a red tongue with scant fur or smooth, peeled, without fur, and fine, rapid pulse

Treatment principles: Supplement and boost the liver and kidneys, enrich yin and cool the blood

Guiding formula: *Da Bu Yuan Jian Jia Jian*

Medicinals: Prepared Radix Rehmanniae (*Shu Di*), Fructus Lycii Chinensis (*Gou Qi Zi*), Tuber Ophiopogonis Japonicae (*Mai Dong*), Fructus Ligustri Lucidi (*Nu Zhen Zi*), Radix Angelicae Sinensis (*Dang Gui*), Fructus Corni Officinalis (*Shan Yu Rou*), Cortex Radicis Moutan (*Dan Pi*), processed Radix Polygoni Multiflori (*Zhi Shou Wu*), Rhizoma Polygonati (*Huang Jing*), Semen Zizyphi Spinosae (*Suan Zao Ren*), Radix Scrophulariae Ningpoensis (*Yuan Shen*), mix-fried Radix Glycyrrhizae (*Zhi Gan Cao*)

Formula explanation: In this formula, prepared Radix Rehmanniae enriches yin and nourishes the blood, supplements the essence and boosts the marrow. The combination of Fructus Lycii Chinensis, Tuber Ophiopogonis Japonicae, Fructus Ligustri Lucidi, processed Radix Polygoni Multiflori, and Rhizoma Polygonati enriches and supplements liver and kidney yin. Radix Angelicae Sinensis nourishes and quickens the blood. Fructus Corni Officinalis supplements the liver and kidneys and astringes the essence. Cortex Radicis Moutan cools the blood and resolves toxins. Radix Scrophulariae Ningpoensis clears heat, resolves toxins, and nourishes yin. Semen Zizyphi Spinosae quiets the spirit and stabilizes palpitations. And Radix Glycyrrhizae regulates and harmonizes the preceding medicinals.

Selected acupuncture/moxibustion points: *Da Zhui* (GV 14)т, *Zu San Li* (St 36)т, *Shen Shu* (Bl 23)т, *Tai Xi* (Ki 3)т, *Tai Chong* (Liv 3)т, & *Gan Shu* (Bl 18)т

Formula rationale: Supplementing *Da Zhui* and *Zu San Li* can supplement and boost qi and blood, boost the essence and engender marrow. *Shen Shu* used in combination with *Gan Shu* supplements and boosts the liver and kidneys. *Tai Xi* is the source point of the kidney channel. Using supplementation technique on it can boost kidney yin and strengthen the brain marrow. Draining *Tai Chong* clears the liver and discharges heat, cools the blood and resolves toxins.

3. *Pi Shen Liang Kui*
Spleen/Kidney Dual Deficiency

Clinical manifestations: A somber white facial complexion, four limbs not warm, low back and knee soreness and weakness, whole body lack of strength, slight edema in the four limbs, food reduced, loose stools, hair falling and fading, a pale, fat tongue, and a deep, fine forceless pulse

Treatment principles: Warm and supplement the spleen and kidneys

Guiding formula: *You Gui Wan Jia Jian*

Medicinals: Prepared Radix Rehmanniae (*Shu Di*), Radix Dioscoreae Oppositae (*Shan Yao*), Fructus Corni Officinalis (*Shan Yu Rou*), Fructus Lycii Chinensis (*Gou Qi Zi*), Radix Astragali Membranacei (*Huang Qi*), Radix Codonopsis Pilosulae (*Dang Shen*), Fructus Psoraleae Corylifoliae (*Bu Gu Zhi*), Herba Epimedii (*Yin Yang Huo*), Gelatinum Cornu Cervi (*Lu Jiao Jiao*), Radix Morindae Officinalis (*Ba Ji Tian*), Caulis Milletiae Seu Spatholobi (*Ji Xue Teng*), Fructus Zizyphi Jujubae (*Da Zao*)

Formula explanation: This formula uses prepared Radix Rehmanniae to supplement the kidneys and fill the essence. Fructus Corni Officinalis, Fructus Psoraleae Corylifoliae, Herba Epimedii, Gelatinum Cornu Cervi, and Radix Morindae Officinalis warm and supplement kidney yang, fill the essence, and engender marrow. Fructus Lycii Chinensis nourishes the liver and enriches the kidneys. Radix Astragali Membranacei, Radix Codonopsis Pilosulae, and Radix Dioscoreae

Oppositae boost the qi and fortify the spleen, greatly supplement the source qi. Caulis Milletiae Jixueteng quickens and supplements the blood. And Fructus Zizyphi Jujubae boosts the qi and nourishes blood, sweetens and mollifies the preceding medicinals.

Selected acupuncture/moxibustion points: *Guan Yuan* (CV 4)▵, *Zu San Li* (St 36)▵, *Da Zhui* (GV 14)▵, *Shen Shu* (GV 14)⊤, & *Pi Shu* (Bl 20)⊤

Formula rationale: Moxaing *Guan Yuan* warms and supplements spleen and kidney yang. *Zu San Li* and *Da Zhui* warm and supplement qi and blood, supplement the essence and engender marrow. *Pi Shu* fortifies the spleen and boosts the qi. Used together, these points warm and supplement spleen and kidney yang to engender marrow.

Note: In clinical practice, Chinese medicinals can be combined together based on differentiation of which kinds of blood cells are low.

For low red blood cells, the commonly used medicinals are: Radix Astragali Membranacei (*Huang Qi*), Radix Codonopsis Pilosulae (*Dang Shen*), Radix Angelicae Sinensis (*Dang Gui*), uncooked Radix Rehmanniae (*Sheng Di*), prepared Radix Rehmanniae (*Shu Di*)Radix Panacis Ginseng (*Ren Shen*), Fructus Lycii Chinensis (*Gou Qi Zi*), Fructus Zizyphi Jujubae (*Da Zao*), Placenta Hominis (*Zi He Che*), Arillus Euphoriae Longanae (*Long Yan Rou*), Gelatinum Corii Asini (*E Jiao*), Gelatinum Cornu Cervi (*Lu Jiao Jiao*).

For low white blood cells, the commonly used medicinals are: Radix Angelicae Sinensis (*Dang Gui*), Radix Astragali Membranacei (*Huang Qi*), Fructus Corni Officinalis (*Shan Yu Rou*), Fructus Lycii Chinensis (*Gou Qi Zi*), Fructus Ligustri Lucidi (*Nu Zhen Zi*), Rhizoma Polygonati (*Huang Jing*), Radix Glehniae Littoralis (*Sha Shen*), Semen Cuscutae (*Tu Si Zi*), Caulis Milletiae Seu Spatholobi (*Ji Xue Teng*), Rhizoma Polygoni Cuspidati (*Hu Zhang*), Herba Epimedii (*Xian Ling Pi*), Fructus Psoraleae Corylifoliae (*Bu Gu Zhi*).

For low blood platelets, the commonly used medicinals are: Gelatinum

Corii Asini (*E Jiao*), Radix Astragali Membranacei (*Huang Qi*), Rhizoma Arachis Hypogaeae (*Hua Sheng Yi*), Herba Agrimoniae Pilosae (*Xian He Cao*), Fructus Ligustri Lucidi (*Nu Zhen Zi*), Rhizoma Polygonati (*Huang Jing*), Fructus Corni Officinalis (*Shan Yu Rou*), Radix Rubiae Cordifoliae (*Qian Cao Gen*), Gelatinum Plastri Testudinis (*Gui Ban Jiao*), Fructus Zizyphi Jujubae (*Da Zao*).

B. *Xiao Hua Xi Tong Fan Ying*
Digestive System Reactions

1. *Gan Wei Bu He*
Liver/Stomach Disharmony

Clinical manifestations: Chest and lateral costal region oppression and fullness, abdomen distended, abdomen painful, belching, burping, nausea, vomiting, loss of regularity of bowel movements, thin, white or slightly yellow tongue fur, and a wiry pulse

Treatment principles: Course the liver and harmonize the stomach, downbear counterflow and stop vomiting

Guiding formula: *Ju Pi Zhu Ru Tang Jia Jian*

Medicinals: Radix Panacis Ginseng (*Ren Shen*), Pericarpium Citri Erythrocarpae (*Ju Pi*), Flos Inulae (*Xuan Fu Hua*), Rhizoma Pinelliae Ternatae (*Ban Xia*), Caulis Bambusae In Taeniis (*Zhu Ru*), Sclerotium Poriae Cocos (*Fu Ling*), Rhizoma Cyperi Rotundi (*Xiang Fu*), Fructus Aurantii (*Zhi Qiao*), uncooked Rhizoma Zingiberis (*Sheng Jiang*), Fructus Zizyphi Jujubae (*Da Zao*), Radix Glycyrrhizae (*Gan Cao*)

Formula explanation: In this formula, Pericarpium Citri Erythrocarpae regulates the qi and harmonizes the middle. Adding Flos Inulae, downbears counterflow and stops vomiting. Radix Panacis Ginseng fortifies the spleen and boosts the qi, boosts the stomach and engenders fluids. Rhizoma Pinelliae Ternatae combined with Caulis Bambusae In Taeniis clears the stomach, downbears counterflow, and stops vomiting.

Rhizoma Cyperi Rotundi and Fructus Aurantii course the liver and rectify the qi, loosen the middle and stop pain. Adding Sclerotium Poriae Cocos fortifies the spleen and aids transportation. Uncooked Rhizoma Zingiberis harmonizes the stomach and stops vomiting. And Radix Glycyrrhizae and Fructus Zizyphi Jujubae boost the qi and harmonize the stomach. Both are adjuvant (ingredients).

Selected acupuncture/moxibustion points: *Zhong Wan* (CV 12)⊥, *Nei Guan* (Per 6)⊥, *Zu San Li* (St 36)⊥, *Tai Chong* (Liv 3)⊥, *Pi Shu* (Bl 20)⊤, & *Gong Sun* (Sp 4)⊥

Formula rationale: Choosing *Zhong Wan*, the front *mu* point of the stomach, and the stomach's sea point, *Zu San Li*, boosts the stomach and harmonizes the middle, downbears counterflow and stops vomiting. *Nei Guan* and *Gong Sun* are eight vessel meeting points. Combining above and below, they are able to rectify the qi and loosen the chest, level surging, downbear counterflow, and stop vomiting. Draining *Tai Chong* courses the liver and regulates the qi. Supplementing *Pi Shu* fortifies the spleen and aids transportation.

2. *Wei Yin Bu Zu*
Stomach Yin Insufficiency

Clinical manifestations: Dry mouth and tongue, nausea and vomiting, loss of appetite, lassitude of the spirit, lack of strength, dizziness, abdominal pain, red tongue with scant fluids, and a fine, rapid pulse

Treatment principles: Boost the stomach and engender fluids, downbear counterflow and stop vomiting

Guiding formula: *Mai Men Dong Tang Jia Jian*

Medicinals: Tuber Ophiopogonis Japonicae (*Mai Dong*), Radix Codonopsis Pilosulae (*Dang Shen*), Semen Oryzae (*Jing Mi*), Rhizoma Pinelliae Ternatae (*Ban Xia*), Herba Dendrobii (*Shi Hu*), Radix Trichosanthis Kirlowii (*Tian Hua Fen*), Rhizoma Anemarrhenae (*Zhi*

Mu), Caulis Bambusae In Taeniis (*Zhu Ru*), Radix Glycyrrhizae (*Gan Cao*)

Formula explanation: Tuber Ophiopogonis Japonicae as the ruling medicinal enriches yin, boosts the stomach, and engenders fluids. It is assisted by Radix Codonopsis Pilosulae and Semen Oryzae which supplement and boost spleen and stomach qi. Thus *jin ye* is automatically engenderd. Rhizoma Pinelliae Ternatae and Caulis Bambusae In Taeniis harmonize the stomach, downbear counterflow, and stop vomiting. Herba Dendrobii, Radix Trichosanthis Kirlowii, and Rhizoma Anemarrhenae enrich yin and boost the stomach, engender fluids and stop thirst. Radix Glycyrrhizae clears heat and disinhibits the throat and also regulates and harmonizes the preceding medicinals.

Selected acupuncture/moxibustion points: *Zu San Li* (St 36)⊤, *Zhong Wan* (CV 12)⊤, *Nei Guan* (Per 6)|, & *San Yin Jiao* (Sp 6)⊤

Formula rationale: Supplementing *Zu San Li* and *Zhong Wan* boosts the stomach and harmonizes the middle, downbears counterflow and stops vomiting. Even supplementation and drainage of *Nei Guan* loosens the chest, rectifies qi, and stops vomiting. Supplementing *San Yin Jiao* boosts the stomach and nourishes yin. The above medicinals used together have the ability to enrich yin and boosts the stomach, downbear counterflow and stop vomiting.

3. *Pi Wei Kui Xu*
Spleen/Stomach Deficiency & Vacuity

Clinical manifestations: Whole body lack of strength, mouth bland and tasteless, no desire for food or drink, abdomen distended, abdomen painful, stools thin and sticky or diarrhea, a pale tongue with thin, white, slimy fur, and a weak, forceless pulse

Treatment principles: Fortify the spleen and boost the qi, harmonize the stomach and disinhibit dampness

Guiding formula: *Xiang Sha Liu Jun Zi Tang Jia Jian*

Medicinals: Radix Codonopsis Pilosulae (*Dang Shen*), Sclerotium Poriae Cocos (*Fu Ling*), Rhizoma Atractylodis Macrocephalae (*Bai Zhu*), Rhizoma Pinelliae Ternatae (*Ban Xia*), Radix Auklandiae (*Mu Xiang*), Pericarpium Citri Reticulatae (*Chen Pi*), Fructus Crataegi (*Shan Zha*), stir-fried Fructus Germinatus Hordei Vulgaris (*Chao Mai Ya*), Radix Glycyrrhizae (*Gan Cao*)

Formula explanation: Radix Codonopsis Pilosulae boosts the qi and fortifies the spleen. It is assisted by Rhizoma Atractylodis Macrocephalae which fortifies the spleen and dries dampness. Sclerotium Poriae Cocos blandly seeps and disinhibits dampness. Rhizoma Pinelliae Ternatae dries dampness. Fructus Amomi (*Sha Ren*) warms the middle and dries dampness, arouses the spleen and harmonizes the stomach. Radix Auklandiae and Pericarpium Citri Reticulatae rectify the qi and fortify the spleen. Adding Fructus Crataegi and Fructus Germinatus Et Praeparatus Hordei Vulgaris fortifies the spleen and harmonizes the stomach, disperses food and transforms stagnation/accumulation. Radix Glycyrrhizae regulates and harmonizes the preceding medicinals. Used together, the above medicinals can boost the qi and fortify the spleen, harmonize the stomach and disinhibit dampness.

For those with severe abdominal pain, add Radix Albus Paeoniae Lactiflorae (*Bai Shao*), Fructus Meliae Toosendanis (*Chuan Lian Zi*), and Rhizoma Corydalis Yanhusuo (*Yan Hu Suo*) to rectify the qi, relax spasm, and stop pain.

Selected acupuncture/moxibustion points: *Pi Shu* (Bl 20)⊤, *Zu San Li* (St 36)⊤, *Zhong Wan* (CV 12)|ᴀ *Yin Ling Quan* (Sp 9)|⊤, & *Tian Shu* (St 25)ᴀ

Formula rationale: Supplementing *Pi Shu* and *Zu San Li* boosts the qi and fortifies the spleen, supplements and boosts qi and blood. Even supplementation and drainage of and adding moxibustion to *Zhong Wan*

warms the center and harmonizes the stomach. Draining *Yin Ling Quan* fortifies the spleen and transforms dampness. Moxaing *Tian Shu* warms, frees, and scatters accumulations, regulates and regulates the stomach and intestines, and stops diarrhea.

C. *Gan Shen Gong Neng Sun Shang*
Liver/Kidney Function Damaged & Injured

1. *Shi Re Nei Yun*
Damp Heat Internally Accumulated

Clinical manifestations: Toxic hepatitis, body and eyes jaundiced, chest and abdominal lumps and fullness, lateral costal aching and pain, nausea and vomiting, aversion to oily, sticky food, tongue fur yellow and slimy, and a wiry, slippery pulse

Treatment principles: Clear heat and disinhibit dampness, resolve toxins and protect the liver

Guiding formula: *Yin Chen Hao Tang Jia Jian*

Medicinals: Herba Artemisiae Capillaris (*Yin Chen Hao*), Fructus Gardeniae Jasminoidis (*Zhi Zi*), Radix Bupleuri (*Chai Hu*), Tuber Curcumae (*Yu Jin*), Sclerotium Poriae Cocos (*Fu Ling*), Fructus Meliae Toosendanis (*Chuan Lian Zi*), Radix Salviae Miltiorrhizae (*Dan Shen*), Radix Angelicae Sinensis (*Dang Gui*), Caulis Akebiae Mutong (*Mu Tong*)

Formula explanation: In this formula, Herba Artemisiae Capillaris clears heat, disinhibits dampness, and recedes jaundice. It is used as the ruling herb. It is assisted by Fructus Gardeniae Jasminoidis and Radix Saussureae Vladimiriae which clear and disinhibit damp heat by expelling damp via urination. Sclerotium Poriae Cocos blandly seeps and disinhibits dampness, fortifies the spleen and aids transportation. Radix Bupleuri, Tuber Curcumae, and Fructus Meliae Toosendanis course the liver, rectify the qi, and stop pain. Radix Salviae

Miltiorrhizae and Radix Angelicae Sinensis nourish and quicken the blood, disperse lumps and scatter nodulation.

Selected acupuncture/moxibustion points: *Da Zhui* (GV 14)⊥, *Zhi Yang* (GV 9)⊥, *Gan Shu* (Bl 18)|, *Yin Ling Quan* (Sp 9)⊥, *Zu San Li* (St 36)⊥, & *Tai Chong* (Liv 3)⊥

Formula rationale: Draining *Da Zhui* clears and discharges yang evils. *Zhi Yang* disinhibits dampness and transforms turbidity to recede jaundice. Even supplementation and drainage of *Gan Shu* courses the liver and regulates the qi. Draining *Yin Ling Quan* clears and disinhibits damp evils. *Zu San Li* fortifies the spleen and aids transportation, harmonizes the middle and disperses distention. *Tai Chong* is chosen to clear and discharge liver/gallbladder damp heat.

2. *Shen Yin Kui Xu*
Kidney Yin Deficiency & Vacuity

Clinical manifestations: Sulfonamide therapy can often cause damage to the kidney function. This may result in intrarenal nephritis or even more severe damage to the kidneys manifesting as oliguria and proteinuria. Low back pain, throat and mouth dry, urination short and frequent or low grade fever, a red tongue, and a fine, rapid pulse

Treatment principles: Enrich yin and boost the kidneys, disinhibit dampness and free stranguria

Guiding formula: *Zhi Bai Di Huang Wan Jia Jian*

Medicinals: Uncooked Radix Rehmanniae (*Sheng Di*), Sclerotium Poriae Cocos (*Fu Ling*), Cortex Radicis Moutan (*Dan Pi*), Rhizoma Alismatis (*Ze Xie*), Radix Dioscoreae Oppositae (*Shan Yao*), Rhizoma Anemarrhenae (*Zhi Mu*), Cortex Phellodendri (*Huang Bai*), Semen Plantaginis (*Che Qian Zi*), Herba Dendrobii (*Shi Hu*), Fructus Corni Officinalis (*Shan Yu Rou*)

Formula explanation: In this formula, Radix Rehmanniae clears heat, nourishes yin, and engenders fluids. Sclerotium Poriae Cocos blandly seeps and disinhibits dampness. Radix Dioscoreae Oppositae boosts the qi, fortifies the spleen, and nourishes yin. Cortex Radicis Moutan clears heat from the yin portion. Rhizoma Alismatis and Semen Plantaginis disinhibit water and free stranguria. Fructus Corni Officinalis enriches yin and supplements the kidneys. Rhizoma Anemarrhenae and Cortex Phellodendri enrich yin and downbear fire, clear heat and moisten dryness. Herba Dendrobii nourishes yin and engenders fluids. Used together, these medicinals are able to enrich and supplement kidney yin, disinhibit dampness and free stranguria.

Selected acupuncture/moxibustion points: *Shen Shu* (Bl 23)⊤, *Guan Yuan* (CV 4)⊤, *Pang Guang Shu* (Bl 28)⊥, *Zu San Li* (St 36)⊤, & *Tai Xi* (Ki 3)⊤

Formula rationale: *Shen Shu* and *Guan Yuan* combined enrich and supplement kidney yin, transform qi and move water. Draining *Pang Guang Shu* clears heat, disinhibits dampness, and frees stranguria. Supplementing *Zu San Li* boosts the qi and fortifies the spleen, cultivates and supplements the postnatal root. *Tai Xi* is the source point of the kidney channel. Supplementing it can enrich and supplement kidney yin and clear empty heat.

If there is damage of the urinary bladder presenting frequent, urgent urination, pain on urination, and hematuria, treatment should consist of clearing heat and resolving toxins, disinhibiting water and freeing stranguria with *Ba Zheng San Jia Jian.*

Medicinals: Caulis Akebiae Mutong (*Mu Tong*), Talcum (*Hua Shi*), Fructus Gardeniae Jasminoidis (*Zhi Zi*), Semen Plantaginis (*Che Qian Zi*), Herba Dianthi (*Ju Mai*), Herba Polygoni Avicularis (*Bian Xu*), Flos Lonicerae Japonicae (*Yin Hua*), Folium Daqingye (*Da Qing Ye*), uncooked Radix Rehmanniae (*Sheng Di*), Rhizoma Imperatae Cyclindricae (*Mao Gen*)

Selected acupuncture/moxibustion points: *Zhong Ji* (CV 3)⊥, *Yin Ling Quan* (Sp 9)⊥, *Pang Guang Shu* (Bl 28)⊥, *Ci Liao* (Bl 32) ⊥ *San Yin Jiao* (Sp 6)⊥

D. *Fang She Xing Yan Zheng* Radiation Inflammation

1. *Re Du Chi Sheng* Hot Toxins Blazing

Clinical manifestations: Skin locally rough, itching or skin thickened, red, swollen, hot, and painful, mouth thirsty, urination scant and red, stools dry and knotted, a red tongue with yellow fur, and a surging, rapid pulse

Treatment principles: Clear heat and resolve toxins

Guiding formula: *Wu Wei Xiao Du Yin Jia Jian*

Medicinals: Flos Lonicerae Japonicae (*Yin Hua*), Fructus Forsythiae Suspensae (*Lian Qiao*), uncooked Radix Rehmanniae (*Sheng Di*), Herba Cum Radice Taraxaci Mongolici (*Pu Gong Ying*), Flos Chrysanthemi Indici (*Ye Ju Hua*), Herba Cum Radice Violae (*Zi Hua Di Ding*), Cortex Radicis Moutan (*Dan Pi*), Radix Angelicae Sinensis (*Dang Gui*), Radix Glycyrrhizae (*Gan Cao*)

Formula explanation: In this formula, Flos Lonicerae Japonicae and Fructus Forsythiae Suspensae clear heat and resolve toxins, disperse swelling and scatter nodulation. They are assisted by Herba Cum Radice Taraxaci Mongolici, Flos Chrysanthemi Indici, and Herba Cum Radice Violae in order to strengthen the clearing of heat and resolution of toxins. Radix Rehmanniae clears heat, nourishes yin, and engenders fluids. Cortex Radicis Moutan resolves toxins and cools the blood. Radix Angelicae Sinensis nourishes and quickens the blood. Radix Glycyrrhizae resolves toxins and also regulates and harmonizes the preceding medicinals.

Selected acupuncture/moxibustion points: *Wei Zhong* (Bl 40)↓, *Qu Chi* (LI 11)⊥, *Da Zhui* (GV 14)⊥, *Zu San Li* (St 36)⊥, & *A Shi* points↓

Formula rationale: *Wei Zhong* and *a shi* points are chosen to bleed in order to clear and discharge blood heat, resolve toxins and scatter nodulation. *Qu Chi* and *Zu San Li* are each the hand and foot *yang ming* sea points. Draining them is able to clear and discharge *yang ming* heat evils. Draining *Da Zhui* recedes heat or fever.

2. *Xie Du Shang Yin*
Evil Toxins Damage Yin

Clinical manifestations: Roughness, thickening, reddening, swelling, or rashes locally on the skin and even difficult to heal skin wounds, essence spirit depression, mouth and tongue dry, sweating, urination short and scant, a red tongue with scant, dry fur, and a fine, rapid pulse

Treatment principles: Cool the blood and resolve toxins, nourish yin and engender fluids

Guiding formula: *Qing Ying Tang Jia Jian*

Medicinals: Uncooked Radix Rehmanniae (*Sheng Di*), Radix Scrophulariae Ningpoensis (*Yuan Shen*), Tuber Ophiopogonis Japonicae (*Mai Dong*), Rhizoma Coptidis Chinensis (*Huang Lian*), Flos Lonicerae Japonicae (*Yin Hua*), Fructus Forsythiae Suspensae (*Lian Qiao*), Fructus Gardeniae Jasminoidis (*Shan Zhi*), Herba Lophatheri Gracilis (*Zhu Ye*), Radix Trichosanthis Kirlowii (*Tian Hua Fen*)

Formula explanation: Radix Rehmanniae, Radix Scrophulariae Ningpoensis, and Tuber Ophiopogonis Japonicae, sweet and cold, clear heat and nourish yin. Rhizoma Coptidis Chinensis, Flos Lonicerae Japonicae, Fructus Forsythiae Suspensae, and Fructus Gardeniae Jasminoidis clear heat, cool the blood, and resolve toxins. Herba Lophatheri Gracilis clears heat and relieves vexation, engenders fluids and stops thirst. Radix Trichosanthis Kirlowii clears heat and engenders fluids, resolves toxins and scatters nodulation. The above medicinals used together have the ability to cool the blood and resolve toxins, nourish yin and engender fluids.

For those with severe inflammation of the oral mucosa with severe aching and pain, add Radix Glehniae Littoralis (*Sha Shen*) and Herba Dendrobii (*Shi Hu*) and more Tuber Ophiopogonis Japonicae (*Mai Dong*), uncooked Radix Rehmanniae (*Sheng Di*), and Radix Scrophulariae Ningpoensis (*Yuan Shen*) to nourish yin, engender fluids, and moisten dryness.

For those with accompanying lung injuries manifesting as fever, cough with phlegm and clotted blood, chest pain, and severe shortness of breath, treatment should clear dryness and moisten the lungs, nourish yin and engender fluids.

Guiding formula: *Qing Zao Jiu Fei Tang Jia Jian*

Medicinals: Folium Mori Albi (*Sang Ye*), Gypsum Fibrosum (*Shi Gao*), Tuber Ophiopogonis Japonicae (*Mai Dong*), Radix Glehniae Littoralis (*Sha Shen*), Semen Pruni Armeniacae (*Xing Ren*), Folium Eriobotryae Japonicae (*Pi Pa Ye*), Bulbus Fritillariae (*Bei Mu*), Herba Agrimoniae Pilosae (*Xian He Cao*), Radix Glycyrrhizae (*Gan Cao*), Gelatinum Corii Asini (*E Jiao*)

Formula explanation: In this formula, Folium Mori Albi lightly diffuses lung dryness. Gypsum Fibrosum clears dry heat from lung metal. Tuber Ophiopogonis Japonicae and Radix Glehniae Littoralis nourish yin, clear heat, and engender fluids. Gelatinum Corii Asini effectively treats yin vacuity (and) lung dryness since it has the ability to enrich yin and moisten dryness. Folium Eriobotryae Japonicae and Semen Pruni Armeniacae clear heat and transform phlegm, stop cough and level asthma. Bulbus Fritillariae moistens the lungs and stops cough, clears and transforms hot phlegm. Herba Agrimoniae Pilosae astringes and stops bleeding. And Radix Glycyrrhizae regulates and harmonizes the preceding medicinals.

Selected acupuncture/moxibustion points: *He Gu* (LI 4)⊥, *Qu Chi* (LI 11)⊥, *Xue Hai* (Sp 10)⊥, *San Yin Jiao* (Sp 6)⊥, & *Tai Xi* (Ki 3)⊤

Formula rationale: Draining *He Gu* and *Qu Chi* diffuses and frees the qi and blood, clears heat and resolves toxins. Draining *Xue Hai* clears and discharges blood heat, cools the blood and resolves toxins. Draining *San Yin Jiao* cools the blood and resolves toxins. And supplementing *Tai Xi* is able to nourish yin and engender fluids.

For those with inflammation of the oral mucosa, add *Lao Gong* (Per 8) with draining technique in order to clear the heart and downbear fire, cool the blood and relieve vexation.

For those with lung damage, add *Fei Shu* (Bl 13) with supplementation technique in order to enrich the lungs and moisten dryness. Also drain *Chi Ze* (Lu 5) to clear and discharge lung heat, transform phlegm and stop coughing.

E. *Zhu She Xing Yan Zheng*
Injection Inflammation

Because of the toxicity of chemotherapeutic drugs, intravenous injection may cause phlebitis and intramuscular injection may cause local aseptic necrosis and secondary inflammation. The pain may be very severe and some patients may even refuse further injections.

Treatment principles: Clear heat and resolve toxins, cool the blood and transform stasis

Guiding formula: *Xian Fang Huo Ming Yin Jia Jian*

Medicinals: Flos Lonicerae Japonicae (*Yin Hua*), Fructus Forsythiae Suspensae (*Lian Qiao*), Fructus Gardeniae Jasminoidis (*Zhi Zi*), Radix Angelicae (*Bai Zhi*), Radix Rubrus Paeoniae Lactiflorae (*Chi Shao*), Spina Gleditschiae Sinensis (*Zao Jiao Ci*), Resina Olibani (*Ru Xiang*), Resina Myrrhae (*Mo Yao*), Caulis Milletiae Jixueteng (*Ji Xue Teng*),

Radix Salviae Miltiorrhizae (*Dan Shen*), Radix Glycyrrhizae (*Gan Cao Shao*)

Selected acupuncture/moxibustion points: *Wei Zhong* (Bl 40)↓, *Qu Chi* (LI 11)⊥, *Da Zhui* (GV 14)⊥, & *A Shi* points↓

III. Immunotherapy & TCM

AIDS is a kind of immunodeficiency disease which is caused by HIV. This is a species of retrovirus which attacks the T-lymphocytes. This virus reproduces in large amounts within the T-lymphocytes which then results in a large scale reduction of these T-cells and hence systemic immunodeficiency. Because of this, methods for regulating and improving immunity are very important in the treatment of AIDS. Unfortunately, (Western) immune regulating drugs, such as 2-interferon, are not very effective. Therefore, Chinese medicinals can be administered to supplement the righteous qi and eliminate evils, thus regulating the immune system and achieving the goal of treating this disease. In recent years, research on Chinese medicinals has progressed greatly, and TCM has been widely applied in clinical practice in the treatment of immunodeficiency and cancer. Modern pharmacological research has demonstrated that Chinese medicinals can improve the immunity of the body. Based on current experience in applying TCM and acupuncture in the clinic, we can say that they not only alleviate symptoms but do also regulate and improve immunity.

According to TCM theory, when the yin and yang of the body are in relative balance, the viscera and bowels function normally. According to modern research, immunity is the balancing of the internal and external environments through immunoprotection and immunosurveillance. Therefore, if there is an imbalance of yin and yang within the body, there will be abnormal immune function and thus the occurrence of disease. In terms of AIDS, those immune system cells which actively provide immune function can be categorized as yang. While those immune system cells which produce the organs and motivate the production of the former cells may be categorized as yin. Further, there is yin within yang and yang within yin. T-helper lymphocytes are yang, but T-inhibitor lymphocytes are yin. These mutually promote and control each other in order to maintain the body's normal state of immunity. However, once there is invasion of the virus, T-helper lymphocytes are injured and the T_4/T_8 ratio is reversed. This causes abnormal immune function and imbalance of yin and yang which can further lead to imbalance of the qi and blood, viscera and bowels, and thence to a series of pathoconditions and patterns. Therefore, treatment should consist of supporting the righteous and securing the root aided by medicinals to eliminate evil and thus improve and regulate the body's immunity.

A. Supporting the Righteous, Securing the Root, & Improving Immunity

It is believed in TCM that, whenever there is an invasion of external evils, there must be an vacuity of righteous qi. Also, invasion by evils can further injure the qi and blood, viscera and bowels. Therefore, the treatment principles should manly consist of supporting the righteous and eliminating evil. This can improve the body's resistance and rebalance the internal and external environments. Modern research has also shown that Chinese medicinals have an ability to help immunity. They can improve and regulate an immune system which has been pathologically affected and even restore it to normal function.

The Chinese medicinals which improve the mononuclear phagocyte system are mostly those having the functions of supplementing the qi and nourishing yin, such as Radix Panacis Ginseng (*Ren Shen*), Radix Astragali Membranacei (*Huang Qi*), Fructificatio Ganodermae Lucidae (*Ling Zhi*), Radix Panacis Quinquifolii (*Xi Yang Shen*), Radix Dioscoreae Oppositae (*Shan Yao*), Rhizoma Atractylodis Macrocephalae (*Bai Zhu*), Rhizoma Polygonati (*Huang Jing*), and Radix Glycyrrhizae (*Gan Cao*). While those which improve humoral immunity mostly fortify the spleen and boost the qi, supplement the kidneys and aid yang, such as Radix Astragali Membranacei (*Huang Qi*), Radix

Codonopsis Pilosulae (*Dang Shen*), Rhizoma Atractylodis Macrocephalae (*Bai Zhu*), Sclerotium Poriae Cocos (*Fu Ling*), Rhizoma Polygonati (*Huang Jing*), Herba Epimedii (*Yin Yang Huo*), Radix Morindae Officinalis (*Ba Ji Tian*), Cortex Cinnamomi (*Rou Gui*), Semen Cuscutae (*Tu Si Zi*), and Rhizoma Curculiginis Orchioidis (*Xian Mao*).

AIDS mainly manifests as deficiency of the cellular immunity of the body. Experiments have shown that the medicinals Radix Panacis Ginseng (*Ren Shen*), Radix Astragali Membranacei (*Huang Qi*), Radix Codonopsis Pilosulae (*Dang Shen*), Rhizoma Atractylodis Macrocephalae (*Bai Zhu*), Radix Dioscoreae Oppositae (*Shan Yao*), Rhizoma Polygonati (*Huang Jing*), Fructufucatio Ganodermae Lucidae (*Ling Zhi*), Cornu Parvum Cervi (*Lu Rong*), prepared Radix Rehmanniae (*Di Huang*), Herba Ecliptae Prostratae (*Han Lian Cao*), and Fructus Schizandrae Chinensis (*Wu Wei Zi*) have the ability to improve T-cells. Also there are some medicinals which improve the transformation of T-cells, such as Radix Astragali Membranacei (*Huang Qi*), Radix Polygoni Multiflori (*Shou Wu*), Gelatinum Corii Asini (*E Jiao*), Semen Cuscutae (*Tu Si Zi*), Fructus Lycii Chinensis (*Gou Qi Zi*), and Fructus Ligustri Lucidi (*Nu Zhen Zi*).

Various supplementing formulas have also proven able to promote cellular immunity. These include *Si Jun Zi Tang, Si Wu Tang, Liu Wei Di Huang Wan,* and *Shen Fu Tang* which all can strengthen phagocytosis. While *Sheng Mai San* can enhance the quality of the T-lymphocytes and improve the body's immunity.

Research on individual medicinals has also proven that Chinese medicinals are very effective in regulating and improving the immunity of the body. It should always be born in mind that the main organs to be supplemented in terms of improving immunity in the treatment of AIDS according to TCM are the lungs, spleen, and kidneys.

1. Kidney Supplementation & Immunity

According to TCM theory, the kidneys are regarded as the prenatal root. They store or treasure source yin and source yang which are the root of yin and yang of the other viscera and bowels. As stated by Zhang Jing-yue, "The yin and yang of all the viscera and bowels are nourished by kidney yin and yang." Modern research has also proven that the kidneys can influence the hypothalamus-pituitary-adrenocortical axis and thus play a part in the maintenance of body immunity. Further, the kidneys govern the bones and the engenderment of marrow. Normal immune cells originate from the multistem cells of the spine. Therefore, supplementing the kidneys can promote the production of bone marrow and immune cells. In the Guangzhou College of TCM Affiliated Hospital, immune deficient patients have been treated with kidney-supplementing medicinals and have shown improvement in the formation rate of T-cells.

Many experiments have proven that Chinese kidney-supplementing medicinals can increase the immune indices of the entire body. Therefore, they can be applied in clinical practice to treat those patients according to their individual cases, whether yin or yang vacuity.

2. Spleen Supplementation & Immunity

The spleen is the source of the engenderment of qi and blood. It governs transportation and transformation of nutrients for the whole body and thus maintains normal organic function. According to modern research, the spleen *vis à vis* immunity is part of an functional unit composed of the anatomical spleen, the organs of blood formation, and the lymphatic system. All of these organs and tissues are the histological basis of the body's immunity. Therefore, the spleen is a very important organ in the maintenance of normal immunity. As Zhang Jing-yue has also said,

> If the spleen qi is vigorous, evils cannot invade. Once there is invasion .
> by external evils, the spleen will be affected.

Thus, in AIDS patients, there is usually spleen vacuity signs and symptoms. Many statistics have shown that spleen supplementing formulas can improve the function of the human body. Formulas such as *Jian Pi Tang, Shen Ling Bai Zhu San,* and *Xiang Sha Liu Jun Zi Tang* can increase the formation of the E-garland and the content of immunoglobulin. It has also been reported by the Shanghai First Hospital that spleen-supplementing decoctions and medicinals have been applied in the treatment of cancer and that, by applying spleen-supplementing and qi-regulating formulas in combination with chemotherapy, the survival rate has been greatly increased. Therefore, spleen supplementation can not only improve the immune function of the body but also reach the goal of controlling the disease.

3. Lung Supplementation & Immunity

It is held in TCM that the lungs govern or rule the qi, the skin, and the defensive qi through the diffusing and dispersing function of the lung qi. In other words, the protective function of the lung qi in Chinese medicine is similar to nonspecific immunity in Western medicine. The occurrence of AIDS is usually caused by weak disease resistance and the invasion of evil qi, and the disease usually shows a number of lung qi vacuity signs and symptoms. Therefore, treatment should mainly consist of supplementing the lungs in cases with lung qi vacuity signs and symptoms. Research has shown that medicinals and decoctions which supplement the lungs can strengthen the resitance of the skin and mucosa. For instance, *Yu Ping Feng San* can improve the body's immunity, relieve opportunistic infections of the upper respiratory tract, relieve symptoms, and shorten the course of such infections.

B. Eliminating Evil & Immunity

Besides supplementation, eliminating evils is also an important treatment principle in the treatment of AIDS. AIDS is usually caused by the invasion of pestilential evils due to vacuity of righteous qi. Therefore, the evil-eliminating method should also be used. The most commonly used methods of eliminating evil include clearing heat and resolving toxins and quickening the blood and transforming stasis. Many researches have shown that evil-eliminating medicinals can improve the body's immunity. For instance, researches have shown that medicinals which quicken the blood and transform stasis can increase body immunity and inhibit pathological immune function. Also, heat clearing and toxin resolving medicinals can not only help the body resist germs and viruses but also stimulate normal immunity and inhibit abnormal immune reactions.

Research on heat-clearing and toxin-resolving medicinals has shown that many medicinals can improve the phagocytosing function of the immune system and increase transformation of lymphocytes as well as the formation of the E-garland. For instance, Flos Lonicerae Japonicae (*Jin Yin Hua*), Herba Andrographidis (*Chuan Xin Lian*), Herba Cum Radice Houttuyniae Cordatae (*Yu Xing Cao*), Radix Sophorae Subprostratae (*Shan Dou Gen*), Flos Chrysanthemi Indici (*Ye Ju Hua*),Rhizoma Paridis Polyphyllae (*Qi Ye Yi Zhi Hua*), Herba Oldenlandiae Diffusae (*Bai Hua She She Cao*), Fructus Forsythiae Suspensae (*Huang Lian*), and Herba Cum Radice Violae (*Zi Hua Di Ding*) can increase phagocytosis within the mononuclear phagocyte system. Herba Cum Radice Taraxaci Mongolici (*Pu Gong Ying*), Herba Cum Radice Violae (*Zi Hua Di Ding*), uncooked Radix Rehmanniae (*Sheng Di*), Radix Scutellariae Baicalensis (*Huang Qin*), Rhizoma Coptidis Chinensis (*Huang Lian*), and Cornu Bubali (*Shui Niu Jiao*) can increase the transformation of lymphocytes. Many formulas which clear heat and resolve toxins, such as *Huang Lian Jie Du Tang*, can also help resist infections and improve the body's immune function.

In addition, those medicinals which quicken the blood and transform stasis or clear heat and resolve toxins can also normalize abnormal immune function. For instance, the heat-clearing, toxin-resolving herb, Radix Scutellariae Baicalensis (*Huang Qin*), can inhibit allergic reactions in the body.

C. Acupuncture/Moxibustion & Immunity

Acupuncture/moxibustion is a very important treatment modality in TCM and is widely applied in clinical practice. It is especially effective in treating certain viral infections and immunodeficiency diseases. Recent research has shown that acupuncture can not only regulate but also improve both the cellular and humoral immunity of the body. Viewing the present state of the treatment of AIDS both in and outside China, acupuncture/moxibustion is widely being applied to improve both the symptoms of this disease and the patients' immunity.

Concerning the nonspecific immunity of the body, acupuncture and moxibustion can improve phagocytosis within the mononuclear phagocyte system. The most commonly chosen points are *Da Zhui* (GV 14), *Zu San Li* (St 36), *He Gu* (LI 4), *Shen Shu* (Bl 23), *Tian Shu* (St 25), and *Shang Ju Xu* (St 37). The effect of acupuncture/moxibustion is closely related to the points chosen and the degree of stimulation. It is reported that puncturing *Da Zhui* (GV 14) with weak stimulation can increase phagocytosis but will decrease phagocytosis with strong stimulation.

Concerning the specific immunity of the body, it has been reported that *Zu San Li* (St 36) can improve the transformation of lymphocytes. In treating kidney vacuity patients with acupuncture/moxibustion, it has been found that patients' T-cells have increased greatly. Moxaing *Da Zhui* (GV 14) and *Fei Shu* (Bl 13) can increase the formation of the E-garland. In treating bacillary dysentery with acupuncture/moxibustion, humoral immunity has been improved with obvious increases in immunoglobulin and nonspecific antibodies. Points having this function include *Zu San Li* (St 36), *Bai Hui* (GV 20), *Da Zhui* (GV 14), *He Gu* (LI 4), *Shen Shu* (Bl 23), and *Guan Yuan* (CV 4).

Acupuncture/moxibustion usually functions by acting on the hypothalamus-hypophysis-adrenocortical axis and thus on the nervous system and humoral immunity. Its most prominent characteristic is that it can regulate in either direction. In other words, it can not only improve hypoimmunity but also normalizes pathological immune function. This fact has provided a useful theoretical basis for the application of acupuncture/moxibustion in clinical practice. In sum, acupuncture/moxibustion can not only regulate but also improve body function.

7

Zhi Liao Ai Zi Bing
Chang Yong Fang Yao

Commonly Used Formulas & Medicinals in the Treatment of AIDS

I. *Yao Wu De Gui Lei*
The Classification of Herbal Medicinals

The medicinals most commonly used for treating AIDS patients are classified according to their pharmacological functions.

A. Chinese Medicinals Which Promote Immune Function

1. Chinese medicinals which promote the mononuclear macro phage system:

Radix Panacis Ginseng (*Ren Shen*), Radix Astragali Membranacei (*Huang Qi*), Radix Codonopsis Pilosulae (*Dang Shen*), Placenta Hominis (*Zi He Che*), Cortex Radicis Acanthopanacis (*Wu Jia Pi*), Herba Epimedii (*Yin Yang Huo*), Rhizoma Atractylodis Macrocephalae (*Bai Zhu*), Fructificatio Ganodermae Lucidae (*Ling Zhi*), Rhizoma

Polygonati (*Huang Jing*), Flos Lonicerae Japonicae (*Jin Yin Hua*), Herba Cum Radice Taraxaci Mongolici (*Pu Gong Ying*), Semen Pruni Persicae (*Tao Ren*), Radix Salviae Miltiorrhizae (*Dan Shen*), Radix Rubrus Paeoniae Lactiflorae (*Chi Shao*), Radix Ligustici Wallichii (*Chuan Xiong*)

2. Chinese medicinals promoting humoral immunity:

Radix Astragali Membranacei (*Huang Qi*), Radix Panacis Ginseng (*Ren Shen*), Rhizoma Atractylodis Macrocephalae (*Bai Zhu*), Sclerotium Poriae Cocos (*Fu Ling*), Rhizoma Polygonati (*Huang Jing*), Herba Epimedii (*Yin Yang Huo*), Radix Morindae Officinalis (*Ba Ji Tian*), Cortex Cinnamomi (*Rou Gui*), Rhizoma Curculiginis Orchioidis (*Xian Mao*), Semen Cuscutae (*Tu Si Zi*), Herba Cistanchis (*Rou Cong Rong*), Radix Scrophulariae Ningpoensis (*Yuan Shen*), Tuber Asparagi Cochinensis (*Tian Dong*), Radix Glehniae Littoralis (*Sha Shen*), Tuber Ophiopogonis Japonicae (*Mai Dong*)

3. Chinese medicinals which promote cellular immunity:

Radix Panacis Ginseng (*Ren Shen*), Radix Astragali Membranacei (*Huang Qi*), Radix Codonopsis Pilosulae (*Dang Shen*), Rhizoma Atractylodis Macrocephalae (*Bai Zhu*), Rhizoma Polygonati (*Huang Jing*), Fructificatio Ganodermae Lucidae (*Ling Zhi*), Radix Dioscoreae Oppositae (*Shan Yao*), Herba Ecliptae Prostratae (*Han Lian Cao*), Semen Cuscutae (*Tu Si Zi*), Gelatinum Corii Asini (*E Jiao*), Herba Epimedii (*Xian Ling Pi*), Radix Angelicae Sinensis (*Dang Gui*), Flos Carthami Tinctorii (*Hong Hua*), Herba Agrimoniae Pilosae (*Xian He Cao*), Radix Salviae Miltiorrhizae (*Dan Shen*), uncooked Radix Rehmanniae (*Sheng Di*), Fructus Ligustri Lucidi (*Nu Zhen Zi*), Flos Lonicerae Japonicae (*Yin Hua*), Fructus Lycii Chinensis (*Gou Qi Zi*), Radix Ligustici Wallichii (*Chaun Xiong*), Radix Albus Paeoniae Lactiflorae (*Bai Shao*), Fructus Schizandrae Chinensis (*Wu Wei Zi*)

4. Chinese medicinals which control immune function:

Radix Glycyrrhizae (*Gan Cao*), Radix Scutellariae Baicalensis (*Huang Qin*), Herba Oldenlandiae Diffusae (*Bai Hua She She Hua*), Semen Pruni Persicae (*Tao Ren*), Fructus Zizyphi Jujubae (*Da Zao*), Herba Artemisiae Apiaceae (*Qing Hao*), Herba Polygoni Perfoliati (*Lie Gong Teng*), Flos Carthami Tinctorii (*Hong Hua*), uncooked Radix Rehmanniae (*Sheng Di*), Radix Bupleuri (*Chai Hu*), Radix Angelicae Sinensis (*Dang Gui*), Rhizoma Alismatis (*Ze Xie*), Fructus Zizyphi Jujubae (*Da Zao*), Caulis Milletiae Seu Spatholobi (*Ji Xue Teng*), Radix Salviae Miltiorrhizae (*Dan Shen*), Herba Leonuri Heterophyllae (*Yi Mu Cao*), Radix Pseudoginseng (*San Qi*), Tuber Curcumae (*Yu Jin*), Rhizoma Sparganii (*San Leng*), Rhizoma Curcumae Zedoariae (*E Zhu*)

5. Anti-allergic Chinese medicinals:

Radix Ledebouriellae Sesloidis (*Fang Feng*), Fructus Schizandrae Chinensis (*Wu Wei Zi*), Radix Gentianae Macrophyllae (*Qin Jiao*), Radix Bupleuri (*Chai Hu*), Fructus Pruni Mume (*Wu Mei*), Radix Stephaniae Tetrandrae (*Han Fang Ji*), Cortex Radicis Moutan (*Dan Pi*), Folium Pyrrosiae (*Shi Wei*), Radix Astragali Membranacei (*Huang Qi*), Placenta Hominis (*Zi He Che*), Flos Daturae Albae (*Yang Jin Hua*), Radix Sophorae Subprostratae (*Shan Dou Gen*), Fructus Immaturus Aurantii (*Zhi Shi*), Fructus Xanthii (*Cang Er Zi*), Radix Glycyrrhizae (*Gan Cao*)

B. Chinese Medicinals Which Combat Disease

1. Chinese medicinals which are anti-viral:

Radix Glycyrrhizae (*Gan Cao*), Herba Cum Radice Violae (*Zi Hua Di Ding*), Radix Trichosanthis Kirlowii (*Tian Hua Fen*), Folium Daqingye (*Da Qing Ye*), Radix Isatidis Seu Baphicacanthi (*Ban Lan Geng*), Flos Lonicerae Japonicae (*Yin Hua*), Fructus Forsythiae Suspensae (*Lian Qiao*), Rhizoma Belamcandae (*She Gan*), Radix Scutellariae Baicalensis (*Huang Qin*), Cortex Phellodendri (*Huang Bai*), Radix Et Rhizoma Rhei

(*Da Huang*), Flos Chrysanthemi Indici (*Ye Ju Hua*), Radix Bupleuri (*Chai Hu*), Radix Lithospermi Seu Arnebiae (*Zi Cao*), Rhizoma Coptidis Chinensis (*Huang Lian*), Herba Andrographidis (*Chuan Xin Lian*), Fructus Xanthii (*Cang Er*), Herba Artemisiae Capillaris (*Yin Chen Hao*), Bulbus Allii Sativi (*Da Suan*), Ramulus Cucumis Sativi (*Huang Gua Gen*)

2. Other Chinese medicinals which combat the causes of disease

a. Broad-spectrum antibiotic medicinals:

Flos Lonicerae Japonicae (*Yin Hua*), Fructus Forsythiae Suspensae (*Lian Qiao*), Folium Daqingye (*Da Qing Ye*), Radix Isatidis Seu Baphicacanthi (*Ban Lan Gen*), Pulvis Indigonis (*Qing Dai*), Cortex Phellodendri (*Huang Bai*), Radix Scutellariae Baicalensis (*Huang Qin*), Herba Cum Radice Violae (*Zi Hua Di Ding*), Herba Cum Radice Taraxaci Mongolici (*Pu Gong Ying*), Herba Patriniae Heterophyllae (*Bai Jiang Cao*), Herba Andrographidis (*Chaun Xin Lian*), Herba Gentianae Scabrae (*Long Dan Cao*), Radix Sophorae Subprostratae (*Shan Dou Geng*), Rhizoma Anemarrhenae (*Zhi Mu*), Fructus Gardeniae Jasminoidis (*Zhi Zi*), Radix Stemonae (*Bai Bu*), Radix Albus Paeoniae Lactiflorae (*Bai Shao*), Cortex Radicis Moutan (*Dan Pi*), Fructus Trichosanthis Kirlowii (*Gua Lou*)

b. Anti-mycotic medicinals:

Rhizoma Coptidis Chinensis (*Huang Lian*), Cortex Phellodendri (*Huang Bai*), Radix Sophorae Flavescentis (*Ku Shen*), Radix Dictamni Dasycarpi (*Bai Xian Pi*), Rhizoma Belamcandae (*She Gan*), Radix Et Rhizoma Rhei (*Da Huang*), Radix Pulsatillae Chinensis (*Bai Tou Weng*), Radix Platycodi Grandiflori (*Jie Geng*), Herba Cum Radice Houttuyniae (*Yu Xing Cao*), Radix Scutellariae Baicalensis (*Huang Qin*), Rhizoma Polygonati (*Huang Jing*), Radix Sophorae Subprostratae (*Shan Dou Geng*), Cortex Pseudolaricis (*Tu Jin Pi*)

c. Anti-spirochetal medicinals:

Folium Daqingye (*Da Qing Ye*), Radix Isatidis Seu Baphicacanthi (*Ban Lang Geng*), Cortex Phellodendri (*Huang Bai*), Fructus Forsythiae Suspensae (*Lian Qiao*), Fructus Gardeniae Jasminoidis (*Zhi Zi*), Herba Andrographidis (*Chuan Xin Lian*), Rhizoma Smilacis Glabrae (*Tu Fu Ling*), Rhizoma Coptidis Chinensis (*Huang Lian*), Radix Scutellariae Baicalensis (*Huang Qin*)

d. Anti-protozoal medicinals:

Radix Pulsatillae Chinensis (*Bai Tou Weng*), Rhizoma Coptidis Chinensis (*Huang Lian*), Radix Scutellariae Baicalensis (*Huang Qin*), Radix Sophorae Flavescentis (*Ku Shen*), Cortex Fraxini (*Qin Pi*), Herba Portulacae Oleraceae (*Ma Chi Xian*), Cortex Phellodendri (*Huang Bai*), Radix Dichroae Febrifugae (*Chang Shan*), Herba Artemisiae Apiaceae (*Qing Hao*), Radix Bupleuri (*Chai Hu*), Radix Sophorae Flavescentis (*Ku Shen*), Herba Agrimoniae Pilosae (*Xian He Cao*)

3. Chinese medicinals which combat cancer:

Bulbus Shancigu (*Shan Ci Gu*), *Qi Shui Xian* (identification unknown), Herba Catharanthi Rosei (*Chang Chun Hua*), *Xi Guo Shu* (identification unknown), Herba Oldenlandiae Diffusae (*Bai Hua She She Cao*), Rhizoma Curcumae Zedoariae (*E Zhu*), Semen Coicis Lachryma-jobi (*Yi Yi Ren*), Sclerotium Polypori Umbellati (*Zhu Ling*), Fructus Trichosanthis Kirlowii (*Gua Lou*), Rhizoma Belamcandae (*She Gan*), Radix Stephaniae Tetrandrae (*Han Fang Ji*), Rhizoma Dioscoreae Bulbiferae (*Huang Yao Zi*), Eupolyphagae Seu Opisthoplatiae (*Tu Bie Chong*), Buthus Martensi (*Quan Chong*), Scolopendra Subspinipes (*Wu Gong*), Hirudo (*Shui Zhi*), Herba Cum Radice Lobeliae Chinensis (*Ban Bian Lian*), Herba Cum Radice Taraxaci Mongolici (*Pu Gong Ying*), Herba Cum Radice Houttuyniae (*Yu Xing Cao*), Radix Salviae Miltiorrhizae (*Dan Shen*), Radix Rubrus Paeoniae Lactiflorae (*Chi Shao*), Radix Pseudoginseng (*San Qi*),

Fructus Psoraleae Corylifoliae (*Bu Gu Zhi*), Herba Sargassii (*Hai Zao*), Herba Scutellariae Barbatae (*Ban Zhi Lian*)

II. *Zhi Liao Ai Zi Bing Chang Yong De Fang Ji* Commonly Used Herbal Formulas in the Treatment of AIDS

A. *Fu Zheng Gu Ben Lei Fang Ji* Formulas Which Support the Righteous & Secure the Root

(The following section in the Chinese original is composed of a listing of various formulas, their ingredients, TCM functions, and indications. Because these formulas are mostly those which have already been discussed in the text above or are well known formulas contained in such standard reference texts as Bensky & Barolet's *Chinese Herbal Medicine: Formulas & Strategies*, we have chosen not to translate this section in its entirety so as not to waste unnecessary paper nor add unnecessary cost to this book. Rather we have chosen to simply list the formulas discussed under this and following similar sections. Based on the brief indications for each formula, practitioners can select from among these lists various guiding formulas which can then be modified to fit their individual patients.)

1. *Yi Guan Jian*: Liver/kidney yin vacuity with liver qi
2. *Shi Quan Da Bu Tang*: Qi & blood vacuity with an element of vacuous cold
3. *Qi Wei Du Qi Wan*: Kidney qi vacuity asthma
4. *Ren Shen Yang Ying Tang*: Dual qi & blood vacuity, heart vacuity
5. *Ba Zhen Tang*: Dual qi & blood vacuity
6. *Da Bu Yuan Jian*: Liver/kidney yin & qi vacuity
7. *Da Bu Yin Wan*: Yin vacuity with flaring of vacuity fire
8. *Tian Wang Bu Xin Dan*: Heart yin & qi vacuity
9. *Liu Jun Zi Tang*: Spleen qi vacuity & dampness

10. *Liu Wei Di Huang Wan*: Kidney yin vacuity
11. *Yu Ping Feng San*: Defensive qi not secured
12. *Zuo Gui Wan*: Kidney yin & essence vacuity
13. *Zuo Gui Yin*: Kidney yin & essence vacuity
14. *You Gui Wan*: Kidney yang & essence vacuity
15. *You Gui Yin*: Kidney yang & essence vacuity
16. *Si Jun Zi Tang*: Spleen qi vacuity & dampness
17. *Si Wu Tang*: Blood vacuity
18. *Sheng Mai San*: Chest qi vacuity
19. *Gui Pi Tang*: Spleen qi & heart blood vacuity
20. *Jia Wei Si Jun Zi Tang*: Spleen qi & kidney essence vacuity
21. *Jia Jian Wei Rui Tang*: Vacuous yin & superficial invasion
22. *Bai He Gu Jin Wan*: Lung yin vacuity with phlegm & heat
23. *An Shen Ding Zhi Wan*: Heart qi vacuity with unstable spirit
24. *Dang Gui Liu Huang Tang*: Yin vacuity & internal heat
25. *Dang Gui Bu Xue Tang*: Blood vacuity
26. *Liu Jun Zi Tang*: Spleen qi vacuity
27. *Qi Ji Di Huang Wan*: Liver/kidney yin vacuity affecting vision
28. *Sha Shen Mai Men Dong Tang*: Lung yin vacuity with lung & stomach heat
29. *Bu Zhong Yi Qi Tang*: Prolapse of central qi
30. *Bu Fei Tang*: Lung qi vacuity
31. *Fu Zi Li Zhong Wan*: Vacuous cold of the spleen/stomach
32. *Hu Qian Wan*: Liver kidney blood & yin vacuity affecting the sinews & bones
33. *He Che Da Zao Wan*: Extreme vacuity of the liver & kidneys
34. *Shi Pi Yin*: Spleen yang vacuity edema
35. *Zhi Bai Di Huang Wan*: Yin vacuity with flaring of empty heat
36. *Jin Gui Shen Qi Wan*: Kidney yang insufficiency
37. *Zhi Gan Cao Tang*: Heart qi & blood vacuity
38. *Shen Fu Tang*: Yang desertion
39. *Shen Su Yin*: Vacuity of the defensive exterior & superficial invasion
40. *Shen Ling Bai Zhu San*: Spleen qi & kidney yin vacuity
41. *Yang Xin Tang*: Heart blood insufficiency

42. *Xiang Sha Liu Jun Zi Tang*: Spleen qi vacuity & dampness complicated by qi stagnation
43. *Qin Jiao Bie Jia San*: Yin vacuity with flaring of empty fire
44. *Zhen Wu Tang*: Spleen yang vacuity edema
45. *Li Zhong Wan*: Vacuity cold of the middle burner
46. *Huang Lian E Jiao Tang*: Heart yin & blood vacuity with flaring fire
47. *Qing Zao Jiu Fei Tang*: Lung dry heat & yin vacuity

B. *Qing Re Jie Du Lei Fang Ji*
Formulas Which Clear Heat & Resolve Toxins

1. *Ba Zheng San*: Damp heat in the lower burner affecting urination
2. *San Ren Tang*: Invasion of external dampness transforming into heat
3. *Qian Jin Wei Jing Tang*: Hot toxins & blood stasis and masses
4. *Xiao Chai Hu Tang*: Hot evils affecting the *shao yang* aspect
5. *Wu Wei Xiao Du Yin*: Hot toxins affecting the skin
6. *Gan Lu Xiao Du Dan*: Hot toxins affecting the mouth & throat
7. *Long Dan Xie Gan Tang*: Damp heat in any of the three burners
8. *Bai Hu Jia Shen Tang*: Evil heat in the *yang ming* aspect
9. *Zhi Bao Dan*: Hot phlegm obstructing the orifices of the heart
10. *An Gong Niu Huang Wan*: Evil heat attacking the pericardium
11. *Zhu Ye Shi Gao Tang*: Lingering heat damaging the qi & yin
12. *Dao Chi San*: Heart heat affecting the small intestine & bladder
13. *Yin Chen Hao Tang*: Damp heat jaundice
14. *Qing Jin Hua Tan Wan*: Hot phlegm in the lungs
15. *Qing Fei Yin*: Lung heat edema
16. *Qing Gu San*: Vacuous yin & bone-steaming fever
17. *Yin Qiao San*: Wind heat invasion
18. *Ge Gen Qin Lian Tang*: Interior heat & external invasion
19. *Xi Jiao Di Huang Tang*: Evil heat entering the blood aspect with stasis/ecchymosis
20. *Xi Huang Wan*: Hot toxins & blood stasis
21. *Bu Ji Xiao Du Yin*: Hot toxins & external wind affecting the hroat
22. *Zheng Ye Tang*: Fluid dryness due to *yang ming* disease

C. *Huo Xue Hua Yu Lei Fang Ji*
Formulas Which Quicken the Blood & Transform Stasis

1. *Hua Ji Wan*: Blood stasis with masses and nodulation
2. *Shao Fu Zhu Yu Tang*: Lower abdominal blood stasis
3. *Xue Fu Zhu Yu Tang*: Uterine blood stasis
4. *Shen Tong Zhu Yu Tang*: Blood stasis causing body pain
5. *Ge Xia Zhu Yu Tang*: Blood stasis below the diaphragm

D. *Ruan Jian San Jie Lei Fang Ji*
Formulas Which Soften the Hard & Scatter Nodulation

1. *Dao Tan Tang*: Dampness, phlegm, & depressive qi
2. *Nei Xiao Lei Li Wan*: Depressive liver qi & phlegm nodulation
3. *Yang He Tang*: Heart yang insufficiency with blood stasis in the chest
4. *Xiao Lei Wan*: Scrofula & lymphadenopathy
5. *Hai Zao Yu Hu Tang*: Depressive qi & phlegm nodulation causing lymphadenopathy
6. *Di Tan Tang*: Aphasia due to wind stike with phlegm obstruction

E. *Qi Ta Fang Ji*
Other Formulas

1. *Tian Ma Gou Teng Yin*: Liver wind due to yin insufficiency
2. *Wu Ling San*: Spleen dampness edema & dysuria
3. *Dan Zhi Xiao Yao San*: Depressive liver fire & spleen vacuity
4. *Zhu Sha An Shen Wan*: Flaring heart fire with unstable spirit
5. *Bao He Wan*: Indigestion due to stagnant food
6. *Ling Gui Zhu Gan Tang*: Spleen yang vacuity with dampness
7. *Chai Hu Shu Gan Tang*: Liver depression qi stagnation with distention & gas

8. *Xiao Yao San*: Liver depression qi stagnation with blood & spleen vacuity
9. *Ling Yang Gou Teng Tang*: Liver wind, phlegm, & heat
10. *Ju Pi Zhu Ru Tang*: Stomach yin vacuity
11. *He Xiang Zheng Qi San*: Invasion of summer heat or external dampness
12. *Zhen Gan Xi Feng Tang*: Liver wind due to blood & yin insufficiency

8

Ai Zi Bing De Yu Fang Ji Tiao Hu

The Prevention & Nursing of AIDS

I. The Prevention of AIDS

AIDS has done great harm to the human race because of both its rapid spread and high death rate. It not only greatly affects the patients' health and causes great suffering to their relatives but seriously threatens surrounding individuals. Therefore, the prevention of this disease is of very great importance. Traditional Chinese Medicine has long treasured the prevention of disease. As early as in the *Nei Jing* there was the idea of *zhi wei bing* or "treating though not diseased." It also emphasized *yu fang wei ran* or "taking preventive measures." In addition, in the *Su Wen* or *Simple Questions*, it says, "The sage does not treat the diseased but the undiseased, nor does he control the rebellious but those who have not yet rebelled." In TCM, the prevention of disease mainly includes two parts, *i.e.*, prevention of the disease in individuals and the prevention of the disease's spread to others.

The onset of AIDS can be looked at from two aspects—that of the righteous qi and that of the evil. Infection by epidemic toxic evils is the outer cause of this disease. While deficiency and emptiness of the viscera and bowels, qi and blood are the internal causes. The outer factors can only function because of these internal causes. Therefore, the prevention of this disease should mainly rest on the treatment of these two factors.

A. The Prevention of Invasion by Epidemic Toxic Evils

Infection by pestilential toxic evils is the main cause of this disease. Therefore, attention should be paid to "avoid toxic qi" in order to prevent invasion by epidemic evils.

B. Cutting Its Routes of Transmission

The AIDS virus mainly spreads through sexual activity, blood transfusion, and blood products. To reduce the spread of infection, the U.S. Department of Health has put forward a number of suggestions which are useful in cutting this disease's routes of transmission.

1. Avoid sexual intercourse with AIDS patients or those who are suspected of having AIDS as well as with drug addicts.

2. Avoid using blood or blood products from members of high risk groups.

3. Apply various tests to identify and dispose of blood and plasma contaminated by the AIDS virus.

4. Doctors should practice extraordinary vigilance when involved with the use of blood products and particularly in the application of blood transfusions. They should encourage patients with prior knowledge of up-coming surgery to store their own blood for future use.

5. Attempts should also be made to test the safety of blood products for hemophiliacs.

C. Controlling HIV Positive Patients

Most of those who are HIV antibody positive do not show any clinical symptoms. Even though they may have a relatively long latency period, they are nonetheless potential sources of infection. Therefore, controlling HIV positive patients is an important part of controlling the spread of AIDS. First, let patients know something about AIDS, such as its cause, routes of transmission, and prevention, so that they can help physicians by controlling their own, everyday personal hygiene, their blood, their secretions and excretions. They should use disposable syringes and should avoid using public showers or shared toothbrushes. Those who are HIV positive must avoid donating blood or other body fluids.

II. Lifestyle

A quiet environment and a peaceful lifestyle are also very important factors for the improvement of disease. Much experience has been accumulated in TCM on this point. In other words, the lifestyle of AIDS patients must not be overlooked either.

A. Environment

A good living environment is good for health. A patient's room should be clean and comfortable. Because of the patient's hypoimmunity, they are usually weak and easily affected by opportunistic infections. Therefore, the room they live in must be very clean, with sufficient sunshine, and well disinfected. Their rooms should also be quiet so that patients can get enough rest. It is believed in TCM that one should adjust along with one's environment. If not, there may be disease or diseases may worsen. AIDS patients usually have very weak resistance. Therefore, they should pay more attention to the changes of each season in order to prevent invasion of external evils. Yang qi and yin essence should be protected to prevent the worsening of this disease.

B. Regular Lifestyle

AIDS patients should arrange their everyday life to keep their living quite regular. Every aspect of human metabolism has its regularity and periodicity. It is held in TCM that people should regulate their lives according to the progression of the four seasons and day and night. This can stabilize the lifestyle and the course of disease. An irregular lifestyle or excessive depression often leads to imbalance of yin and yang, qi and blood and thus worsen the case.

C. Balancing Work & Rest

Either extreme work or extreme rest may cause undesirable, abnormal function of the qi and blood, viscera and bowels. In the *Nei Jing* there is the saying, "Extreme taxation exhausts the qi." That means that overworking may not only weaken the function of the viscera and bowels but also exhaust the qi of the spleen/stomach, kidneys, and lungs. However, if the patient always rests in fear of overworking, the qi and blood and viscera and bowels may also weaken due to lack of vitality. As it is said, "Prolonged lying damages the qi." Therefore, balancing work or activity with rest should also be an important part of the treatment plan. Along with sufficient rest, appropriate exercises should also be applied, such as *Tai Ji Quan*, *Qi Gong*, and relaxed walking. These can promote the function of the viscera and bowels as well as of the qi and blood.

D. Restricting Sexual Activity

The occurrence of this disease is usually caused by abnormal sexual activity which exhausts the kidney essence which, in turn, allows invasion of evil toxins. If patients continue to indulge in sensual pleasure, this may further exhaust kidney essence and source qi. What's more, sexual activity may also transmit the pestilential evils. Therefore, patients should restrict their desires in order to conserve their essence and maintain sufficient source qi, thus controlling their disease.

III. Dietary Therapy

Dietary therapy is an important method for maintaining the vitality of the body. It is necessary to take enough protein and calories in a balanced diet to keep up one's health. It is believed in TCM that the function of the viscera and bowels is supported by the nutritive essence from food. As stated in the *Nei Jing*, "All people live on food." Because of the invasion of evil qi, the body of AIDS patients is usually weak. In addition, to overcome disease and recover from its injuries, sufficient nutrition must be supplied to the body. Hence the importance of appropriate food intake.

One of the characteristics of this disease is progressive emaciation and weight loss. To make matters worse, the disease itself and the side effects of its treatment may also cause poor appetite. Therefore, patients are usually only half hungry. This may result in a pernicious cycle leading to poor formation of qi and blood which, in turn, affects the survival of the patient. Thus, active steps should be taken to achieve a sufficient supply of nutrients. The following measures can be taken to improve the patient's appetite.

A. One should eat frequent, small amounts of food. This can not only supply patients with sufficient amounts of food but also help in promoting the appetite.

B. One should eat appropriate high calorie foods, such as meat and eggs, to make up for poor food intake.

C. One should change the types of food eaten frequently, especially their color, smell, and flavor, in order to arouse the patient's appetite.

D. One should try to keep a good mood when eating. Patients should eat with their relatives or other patients together to create a warm atmosphere so as to also increase their appetite.

It is also held in TCM that some foods should be especially avoided.

A. One should restrict greasy, fried, hot, peppery foods as well as alcohol.

B. For those patients with fever, foods which are warm or hot in nature should be restricted and especially those foods with hot flavor, such as ginger, garlic, and chili peppers. These can worsen the disease.

C. In chronic cases, viscera and bowel function is usually weak and there is poor function of stomach qi. Therefore, greasy, cold, and raw foods should be restricted, nor should one overeat or overdrink in case stomach qi be damaged and the disease worsen.

In sum, patients should be given, frequent, small amounts of various kinds of delicious food. One should try to avoid greasy food to protect the stomach qi. Also, patients should be persuaded neither to be picky nor to overeat. Those nutritious and light foods, such as mushroom and black fungus, which can also improve the body's immunity, should be taken frequently.

General Index

A

abdominal distention 63, 67, 100, 106, 112, 113, 150
abdominal distention after eating 100
abdominal distention and fullness 63
abdominal masses 16, 23, 175
abdominal pain 6, 107, 110, 114, 201, 203
acid regurgitation 113
agitation 57, 69, 77, 88, 96, 107, 157
AKP 174
alkaline phosphatase 174
allergic reaction 7
An Gong Niu Huang Wan 58, 226
An Shen Ding Zhi Wan 140, 225
anemia 99, 194
anger 21
angered, easily 157
antibiotic medicinals 222
anxiety 69, 134
apathy 7
aphasia 28, 227
ARC 6-8, 26, 51, 52, 78, 91, 99, 105, 117, 141
arthralgia 6
Aspergillus 177
asthenia 99, 100
asthma 24, 62, 84, 85, 123-126, 128, 129, 183, 184, 209, 224
asymptomatic latency period 7
autoimmune disease 7
awakened, easily 137, 139, 140
AZT 10, 11, 194

B

Ba Zhen Tang 65, 101, 176, 195, 224
Ba Zheng San 178, 206, 226
bacillary dysentery 217
Bai He Gu Jin Tang 103, 151
Bai He Gu Jin Wan 225
Bai Hu Jia Ren Shen Tang 57
Bai Hu Jia Shen Tang 226

Bao He Wan 113, 227
basement membrane deposits 177
ben 31, 36, 224
bian bing 30, 31
bian bing lun zhi 30
bian zheng 15, 29-31, 35, 45, 89, 91
Bian Zheng Lu 15
bian zheng lun zhi 30
biao 14, 31, 131
bing ji 13, 17, 92
Bing Peng San 156
bing yin 13, 17, 92
bleeding 14, 49, 83, 97, 98, 102, 127, 149, 150, 154, 157, 161, 163, 165, 209
blindness 168, 169, 172
blood network vessels 14, 19
blood stasis 18, 21-24, 28, 42, 43, 79, 80, 93, 165, 166, 169, 170, 174, 175, 179, 181, 185, 226, 227
bodily fatigue 148
body cold 110, 183, 184
body feels hot 153
body resistance 25, 39, 79
bone marrow 193-195, 214
borborygmus 67, 70, 106
brain cortex 134
breath, shortness of 8, 27, 55, 60, 61, 65, 66, 88, 94, 100, 101, 114, 124, 133, 140, 146, 152, 155, 173, 183, 185, 209
breath, shortness of, on exertion 55
bronchi 123
Bu Fei Tang 60, 127, 225
Bu Ji 23, 112, 226
bu ji bu na 112
Bu Ji Xiao Du Yin 226
bu mei 135
bu nei bu wai yin 18
bu shi shi 112
bu si shi 112
Bu Zhong Yi Qi Tang 66, 70, 94, 155, 225
burping 200

E

eat or drink, inability to 122
eating but without taste 113
eating, distention after 100, 114
eczema 160
edema in the feet 167
edema of the body and limbs 95
eight principles 30
eliminating evil 33-36, 41, 48, 56, 78, 212, 215
elimination 35, 41
emaciation 14, 15, 27, 52, 57, 63, 66, 70, 77, 79, 88, 93, 94, 99-102, 104, 109, 113, 128, 146, 167, 175, 176, 179, 233
emesis 35
emotional depression 67, 79, 112, 115, 142, 187
encephalitis 9
endocarditis 181
enzymes 37
epigastric and abdominal lumps and fullness 70
epiglottis 148
epilepsy 10, 17, 24, 28, 188, 189
epistaxis 97
eructation 113
essence spirit depression 208
evil qi 17, 18, 20, 24-26, 28, 53, 215, 233
extremities and body tired and weary 159
extremities weak 155
eyes, deviated mouth and 86
eyes dry and grating 171
eyes red 57

F

facial complexion, dark 79, 176
facial complexion, pale white 65, 74, 89, 146
facial complexion, somber white 70, 94, 110, 120, 195, 198
facial edema 74
fang lao 22

fatigue 6, 14, 27, 46, 52, 70, 94, 101, 148, 159
fear 21, 26, 27, 53, 60, 119, 131, 134, 135, 232
fear of wind 53, 60, 131
feces clear and thin or watery 110
feet, edema in the 167
fever 6-9, 15, 26, 27, 52, 53, 55, 57-61, 76, 77, 82, 91-96, 98, 99, 102, 106, 107, 111, 119, 124, 126-128, 130, 132, 133, 137, 138, 143, 148, 149, 151, 157, 168, 196, 205, 208, 209, 226, 234
fever aggravated by taxation 55
fever and chills 15
fever in the afternoon or night 98
fever, intermittent low 8
fever not relieved by sweating 57
fever sometimes high, sometimes low 95
flowers dancing in the air 171
forgetful 71
four diagnoses 30, 192
fright 21, 49, 70
fu qi wen bing 14
fu zheng 33, 36, 49, 51, 224
fu zhong xi yi 191
Fu Zi Li Zhong Tang 74
fungal infections 152

G

Gan Lu Xiao Du Dan 82, 96, 226
Gan Mai Da Zao Tang 189
Ge Gen Qin Lian Tang 108, 226
Ge Xia Zhu Yu Tang 80, 175, 227
glycyrrhizin 10, 48
grief 21
Gu Ling Yi Jian 17
Guangzhou College of TCM Affiliated Hospital 214
Gui Pi Tang 69, 136, 225
Gui Zhi Gan Cao Long Gu Mu Li Tang 183

H

Hai Zao Yu Hu Tang 227
hair falling and fading 71, 198
hallucinations 10
hands and feet chilly or not warm 69, 74
harmonization 35
He Che Da Zao Wan 225
He Che Zai Zao Wan 72
headache 10, 95, 119
heart vexation 67, 95, 133, 138, 139, 154
heat in the hands, feet, and heart 53, 137
hematemesis 97
hematuria 206
hemiplegia 24
hemophiliacs 4, 230
hemorrhage 26, 97, 168, 170
hemorrhage, subcutaneous purpuric 97
Herpes mucosae 8
Herpes simplex 8, 10, 152, 157, 186
Herpes zoster virus 9
hiccups 115
hidden qi warm disease 14
HIV 1, 5, 18, 20, 25, 30, 51, 191, 211, 231
Hodgkin's disease 10
homosexual activities 3
hormone levels 37
HTLV III 5
Hu Qian Wan 225
Hua Ji Wan 176, 227
Huang Lian Jie Du Tang 216
human immune deficiency virus 5, 46
Hunan Medical College Affiliated Hospital 194
Huo Xiang Zheng Qi San 106, 119
hypoimmunity 5, 13, 20, 43, 152, 218, 231
hyposexuality 7

I

ideas not clear 77
immune system depression 123
immunoglobulin 37, 215, 217
immunoprotection 211

immunosurveillance 211
impotence 7, 70, 73
inability to eat or drink 122
inability to walk 15
infectious epidemic disease 14
injection 11, 25, 194, 210
insomnia 47, 53, 128, 134, 135, 187, 189
isopropyl inosine 10
itching 8, 69, 74, 83, 157, 160-164, 207
itching sometimes during the day, sometimes at night 163

J, K

jaundiced, body and eyes 204
jaw, scrofulous lumps under the 81
Jia Jian Wei Rui Tang 225
Jia Wei Si Jun Zi Tang 62, 225
Jian Pi Tang 215
Jie Du Hua Yu Wan 166
Jin Gui Shen Qi Wan 70, 225
Jin Gui Yao Lue 14
Jin Huang San 159
Jing Yue Quan Shu 22, 40, 92
joints, soreness in the 7
joy 21
Ju Pi Zhu Ru Tang 122, 200, 228
Kaposi's sarcoma 2, 5-10, 79, 165, 174, 177, 181
ke chuan 17, 123
keratitis 10

L

larynx 148, 149, 152
lassitude of the spirit 55, 61-63, 65, 66, 71, 100, 102, 109, 114, 131, 135, 144, 146, 155, 173, 179, 181, 183, 189, 201
LAV 5
legs weak 74
lentinan 10
leukoplakia 152
Li Zhong Wan 110, 225, 226
Liang Ge San 153

O

oliguria 205
oral apathae 152
oral candidiasis 9
oral mucosa 152, 165, 209, 210

P

palpitations 14, 53, 55, 69, 85, 88, 93, 94, 101, 121, 135, 137, 163, 173, 181-185, 195-197
PCP 5, 8, 9
pericarditis 181
pericardium 58, 70, 94, 97, 116, 154, 181, 226
peripheral nerves 157
perspiration, spontaneous 55, 60-62, 66, 70, 94, 130, 131, 133
pestilence 14
pestilential qi 18
pestilential toxins 19, 105
phagocytosis 38, 213, 216, 217
phlegm 15-18, 23, 24, 28, 32, 34, 43, 44, 53-56, 58, 60, 61, 79, 81, 82, 84-87, 102, 103, 118, 121, 122, 124-129, 142-147, 149, 151, 154, 165, 168, 169, 171, 174, 187-189, 209, 210, 225-228
phlegm mixed with blood 61
phlegm nodulation 24, 43, 227
phlegm turbidity 24, 34, 44, 79, 81, 82, 87, 124, 142, 144, 165, 169, 174, 187, 188
phlegm wheezing in the throat 85
physically weak 47
placenta 3, 4, 72, 173, 199, 219, 221
pleura 123
Pneumocystis bacteria 10
Pneumocystis carinii pneumonia 2, 5, 8
pneumonia, interstitial 9
premature ejaculation 53
professional transmission 4
prostitutes 3
proteinuria 205
pruritus 160

Pseudomonas aeruginosa 147
pulmonary lobes 123
purgation 35

Q

qi counterflow 128
qi gong 232
qi hua 84
Qi Ju Di Huang Wan 172
Qi Wei Du Qi Wan 224
Qian Jin Fang 52
Qin Jiao Bie Jia San 226
Qing Dai Gao 159
Qing Fei Yin 226
Qing Gu San 226
Qing Hao Bie Jia Tang 93
Qing Jin Hua Tan Tang 126
Qing Yan Li Ge Tang 150
Qing Ying Tang 58, 97, 208
Qing Zao Jiu Fei Tang 61, 209, 226
qu xie 33

R

radiation therapy 192, 193
rash 7
re chuang 157
rectal lingulate carcinoma 10
rectal mucosa 3
rectal squamous carcinoma 10
Ren Shen Gui Pi Wan 47
renal failure 177
restlessness 57, 67, 69, 196
retinal periphlebitis 168
retrovirus 3, 5, 186, 211
reverse transcriptase 11
ribavirin 10
righteous qi 16, 19, 24-28, 31-34, 36, 38, 46, 50, 52, 53, 57, 67, 79, 105, 148, 153, 157, 165, 174, 180, 181, 193, 211, 212, 215, 229

S

saliva 3, 121
Salmonella 105
San Ren Tang 169, 226
scrofula 15, 16, 18, 24, 28, 43, 54, 56, 82, 141-147, 227
scrofulous lumps under the jaw 81
seborrheic dermatitis 8, 160
seminal emission 53, 70, 73, 104, 138, 197
sexual organs 3
sexual transmission 3
Sha Shen Mai Dong Tang 128
Shanghai First Hospital 215
Shao Fu Zhu Yu Tang 227
she cuan chuang 157
Shen Fu Tang 89, 129, 213, 225
Shen Su Yin 56, 225
Shen Tong Zhu Yu Tang 227
Sheng Ling Bai Zhu San 38
Sheng Ma Xiao Du Yin 167
Sheng Mai San 61, 89, 133, 213, 225
Shi Pi Yin 225
Shi Quan Da Bu Tang 224
shortness of breath 8, 27, 55, 60, 61, 65, 66, 88, 94, 100, 101, 114, 124, 133, 140, 146, 152, 155, 173, 183, 185, 209
shortness of breath on exertion 55
Si Huang Gao 159
Si Jun Zi Tang 47, 51, 55, 60, 62, 65, 69, 71, 100, 109, 147, 173, 177, 213, 225
Si Wu Tang 147, 164, 173, 177, 213, 225
sighing 49, 67, 139
skin flushed red 157
skin locally rough 207
skin rashes 8, 26, 58, 59, 160, 165
skin thickened 207
skin tubercles 165
sleep, lack of 61, 67, 69, 75, 77, 101
spasms and convulsions 86, 87
speak, disinclination to 60, 61, 94, 100, 114, 152, 155
sperm 3, 19
spirit, lassitude of the 55, 61-63, 65, 66,
71, 100, 102, 109, 114, 131, 135, 144, 146, 155, 173, 179, 181, 183, 189, 201
Staphylococcus 147, 152
stomach and intestinal tract dysfunction 112
stomachache 26
stools, blood in the 14, 97
Streptococcus 147, 152
Su Wen 14, 15, 18, 25, 26, 31, 36, 229
subcutaneous nodules of varying size 81
Sulfonamide therapy 205
supporting the righteous 32-36, 41, 48, 78, 212
suramin 10
sweating 7, 52, 57, 61, 66, 89, 127, 130-134, 208

T

T4 helper lymphocytes 5
T4/T8 ratio 46, 212
T8 inhibitor lymphocytes 5
tai ji quan 232
The Analysis of Weakness 38
thirst 53, 57, 64, 92, 97, 98, 106, 107, 117, 123, 124, 129, 131, 149, 153, 154, 157, 159, 171, 202, 208
throat and larynx red and swollen or ulcerated 149
throat, sore 7, 53, 82, 124, 147-149
throat, sound of phlegm in the 127
thrush 7, 9, 26, 152-155
Tian Wang Bu Xin Dan 137, 224
tinnitus 70, 71, 75, 77, 88, 104, 132, 137, 138, 172, 196
tonsils 147, 148
toxic qi 15, 25, 52, 230
toxic reaction 7
toxoplasmatic retinitis 10
toxoplasmosis 9, 79
transaminase 174
transient symptomatic stage 6
treatment methods 31, 35, 36, 60, 194
tubercles all over the lower limbs 166

tumors and masses 80
tumors, malignant 7

U

U.S. Department of Health 230
ulcers and exudation 159
unconsciousness 24, 85, 187
urethritis 178
urinary pain 178
urinary urgency 178
urination burning hot 178

V

vacuity taxation 14, 15, 27, 28, 61, 62
vacuity vexation 128
vertigo 24, 74, 86
vertigo, severe 86
vexation 57, 67, 69, 77, 86, 88, 92, 95-97, 107, 116, 128, 133, 134, 138, 139, 141, 143, 154, 155, 157, 189, 208, 210
vexatious heat in the five centers 103
Vibrio jejuni 105
viral evils 14, 19, 20, 22, 25, 34, 38, 46
viral syndrome, acute nonspecific 7
vision, dimming and blurring of 168
vision unclear 72
vocal chords 148
voice, feeble 27, 66, 70
vomiting 63, 64, 86, 95, 99, 106, 107, 110, 117-123, 200-202, 204

W

Wai Ke Zheng Zong 16
Wai Sheng Bao Jian 16
wai yin 18
walk, inability to 15
warming 35, 39, 184
water blisters after scratching 162
water passageways 23, 178-180
weakness 7, 8, 14, 16, 36, 38, 43, 47, 53,
70, 75, 77, 79, 86, 92, 101, 104, 105, 109, 110, 118, 124, 130, 138, 172, 197, 198
weals and rashes 161, 162
weary 55, 57, 120, 151, 152, 159, 176, 195
wei biao 131
Wei Ling Tang 159
Wei Ru Tang 54
weight loss 6-8, 46, 99, 111, 233
wen bing 14
wen yi 14, 18
Wen Yi Lun 18
wheezing 85, 123, 127
wind, fear of 53, 60, 131
work, unable to 55, 57, 152
worry 21, 22, 134
Wu Ling San 227
Wu Wei Xiao Du Yin 207, 226

X

Xi Huang Wan 145, 226
Xi Jiao Di Huang Tang 226
Xi Lei San 156
Xiang Bei Yang Ying Wan 146
Xiang Sha Liu Jun Zi Tang 38, 203, 215, 226
Xiao Ban Xia Tang 121
Xiao Chai Hu Tang 50, 226
Xiao Feng San 161
Xiao Jin Dan 147
Xiao Lei Wan 227
Xiao Luo Wan 81
Xiao Yao San 67, 115, 227, 228
Xue Fu Zhu Yu Tang 98, 171, 227

Y

Yang He Tang 227
Yang Xin Tang 189, 225
Yang Yin Qing Fei Tang 54
Yi Gong San 114
Yi Guan Jian 77, 224
Yi Wei Tang 116

Yi Xue Gang Mu 17
Yin Chen Hao Tang 204, 226
Yin Qiao San 125, 226
Yong Ke Chuan Xin De Ji 17
You Gui Wan 73, 74, 198, 225
You Gui Yin 225
yu fang wei ran 229
Yu Ping Feng San 55, 131, 215, 225

Z

Zhen Gan Xi Feng Tang 86, 228
Zhen Wu Tang 184, 226
Zheng Ye Tang 226
Zheng Zhi Hui Bu 118
Zhi Bai Di Huang Wan 76, 154, 205, 225
Zhi Bao Dan 226
Zhi Gan Cao Tang 88, 182, 225
Zhong Zang Jing 18
Zhu Bing Yuan Hou Lun 16
Zhu Huang San 156
Zhu Sha An Shen Wan 227
Zhu Ye Shi Gao Tang 226
Zhuan Dai Dan 187
Zuo Gui Wan 75, 225
Zuo Gui Yin 225

OTHER BOOKS ON CHINESE MEDICINE AVAILABLE FROM BLUE POPPY PRESS

1775 Linden Ave, Boulder, CO 80304
For ordering 1-800-487-9296
PH. 303\447-8372 FAX 303\447-0740

STICKING TO THE POINT: A Rational Methodology for the Step by Step Formulation & Administration of an Acupuncture Treatment by Bob Flaws ISBN 0-936185-17-1 $16.95

ENDOMETRIOSIS, INFERTILITY AND TRADITIONAL CHINESE MEDICINE: A Laywoman's Guide by Bob Flaws ISBN 0-936185-14-7 $9.95

THE BREAST CONNECTION: A Laywoman's Guide to the Treatment of Breast Disease by Chinese Medicine by Honora Lee Wolfe ISBN 0-936185-61-9, $9.95

NINE OUNCES: A Nine Part Program For The Prevention of AIDS in HIV Positive Persons by Bob Flaws ISBN 0-936185-12-0 $9.95

THE TREATMENT OF CANCER BY INTEGRATED CHINESE-WESTERN MEDICINE by Zhang Dai-zhao, trans. by Zhang Ting-liang & Bob Flaws, ISBN 0-936185-11-2, $18.95

A HANDBOOK OF TRADITIONAL CHINESE DERMATOLOGY by Liang Jian-hui, trans. by Zhang Ting-liang & Bob Flaws, ISBN 0-936185-07-4 $15.95

A HANDBOOK OF TRADITIONAL CHINESE GYNECOLOGY by Zhejiang College of TCM, trans. by Zhang Ting-liang, ISBN 0-936185-06-6 (4nd edit.) $22.95

PRINCE WEN HUI'S COOK: Chinese Dietary Therapy by Bob Flaws & Honora Lee Wolfe, ISBN 0-912111-05-4, $12.95 (Published by Paradigm Press, Brookline, MA)

THE DAO OF INCREASING LONGEVITY AND CONSERVING ONE'S LIFE by Anna Lin & Bob Flaws, ISBN 0-936185-24-4 $16.95

FIRE IN THE VALLEY: The TCM Diagnosis and Treatment of Vaginal Diseases by Bob Flaws ISBN 0-936185-25-2 $16.95

HIGHLIGHTS OF ANCIENT ACUPUNCTURE PRESCRIPTIONS trans. by Honora Lee Wolfe & Rose Crescenz ISBN 0-936185-23-6, $14.95

ARISAL OF THE CLEAR: A Simple Guide to Healthy Eating According to Traditional Chinese Medicine by Bob Flaws, ISBN #-936185-27-9 $8.95

PEDIATRIC BRONCHITIS: Its Cause, Diagnosis & Treatment According to Traditional Chinese Medicine trans. by Gao Yu-li and Bob Flaws, ISBN 0-936185-26-0 $15.95

AIDS & ITS TREATMENT ACCORDING TO TRADITIONAL CHINESE MEDICINE by Huang Bing-shan, trans. by Fu-Di & Bob Flaws, ISBN 0-936185-28-7 $24.95

ACUTE ABDOMINAL SYNDROMES: Their Diagnosis & Treatment by Combined Chinese-Western Medicine by Alon Marcus, ISBN 0-936185-31-7 $16.95

MY SISTER, THE MOON: The Diagnosis & Treatment of Menstrual Diseases by Traditional Chi-

nese Medicine by Bob Flaws, ISBN 0-936185-34-1, $24.95

FU QING-ZHU'S GYNE-COLOGY trans. by Yang Shou-zhong and Liu Da-wei, ISBN 0-936185-35-X, $22.95

FLESHING OUT THE BONES: The Importance of Case Histories in Chinese Medicine trans. by Charles Chace. ISBN 0-936185-30-9, $18.95

CLASSICAL MOXIBUSTION SKILLS in Contemporary Clinical Practice by Sung Baek, ISBN 0-936185-16-3 $12.95

THE MEDICAL I CHING: Oracle of the Healer Within by Miki Shima, OMD, ISBN 0-936185-38-4, $19.95

MASTER TONG'S ACUPUNC-TURE: An Ancient Lineage for Modern Practice, trans. and commentary by Miriam Lee, OMD, ISBN 0-936185-37-6, $19.95

A HANDBOOK OF TCM UROL-OGY & MALE SEXUAL DYSFUNCTION by Anna Lin, OMD, ISBN 0-936185-36-8, $16.95

MASTER HUA'S CLASSIC OF THE CENTRAL VISCERA by Hua Tuo, ISBN 0-936185-43-0, $21.95

THE HEART & ESSENCE OF DAN-XI'S METHODS OF TREATMENT by Xu Dan-xi, trans. by Yang Shou-zhong, ISBN 0-926185-49-X, $21.95

STATEMENTS OF FACT IN TRADITIONAL CHINESE MEDICINE by Bob Flaws, ISBN 0-936185-52-X, $12.95

IMPERIAL SECRETS OF HEALTH & LONGEVITY by Bob Flaws, ISBN 0-936185-51-1, $9.95

THE SYSTEMATIC CLASSIC OF ACUPUNCTURE & MOXIBUS-TION (Jia Yi Jing) by Huang-fu Mi, trans. by Yang Shou-zhong and Charles Chace, ISBN 0-936185-29-5, $79.95

CHINESE MEDICINAL WINES & ELIXIRS by Bob Flaws, ISBN 0-936185-58-9, $18.95

THE DIVINELY RESPONDING CLASSIC: A Translation of the Shen Ying Jing from Zhen Jiu Da Cheng, trans. by Yang Shou-zhong & Liu Feng-ting ISBN 0-936185-55-4, $15.95

PAO ZHI: An Introduction to Processing Chinese Medicinals to Enhance Their Therapeutic Effect, by Philippe Sionneau, ISBN 0-936185-62-1, $34.95

THE BOOK OF JOOK: Chinese Medicinal Porridges, An Alternative to the Typical Western Breakfast, by Bob Flaws, ISBN0-936185-60-0, $16.95

SHAOLIN SECRET FORMULAS for the Treatment of External Injuries, by De Chan, ISBN 0-936185-08-2, $18.95

AGING & BLOOD STASIS: A New Approach to TCM Geriatrics, by Yan De-xin, ISBN 0-936185-63-5, $21.95

CHINESE MEDICAL PALM-ISTRY: Your Health in Your Hand, by Zong Xiao-fan & Gary Liscum, ISBN 0-936185-64-3, $15.95

THE SECRET OF CHINESE PULSE DIAGNOSIS by Bob Flaws, ISBN 0-936185-67-8, $17.95

LOW BACK PAIN: Care & Prevention with Traditional Chinese Medicine by Douglas Frank, ISBN 0-936185-66-X, $9.95

A COMPENDIUM OF TCM PATTERNS & TREATMENTS by Bob Flaws & Daniel Finney, ISBN 0-936185-70-8, $29.95

ACUPUNCTURE AND MOXIBUSTION FORMULAS & TREATMENTS by Cheng Dan-an, trans. By Wu Ming, ISBN 0-936185-68-6, $22.95

THE TREATMENT OF DISEASE IN TCM: Diseases of the Head & Face Including Mental/Emotional Disorders by Philippe Sionneau & Lü Gang, ISBN 0-936185-69-4, $21.95